IN SEARCH OF MY HUSBAND'S MIND

by

WINNIE HIRSCH

IN SEARCH OF MY HUSBAND'S MIND

by

WINNIE HIRSCH

Pathfinder Publishing
Ventura, California

Copyright © 1997 by Winnie Hirsch

Pathfinder Publishing of California
458 Dorothy Avenue
Ventura, CA 93003
(805) 642-9278

Library of Congress Cataloging-in-Publication Data

Hirsch, Winnie, 1917-
    In search of my husband's mind / by Winnie Hirsch.
       p.   cm.
    ISBN 0-934793-64-6
    1. Hirsch,, Monroe J.--Health. 2. Medicine--Malpractice.
    3. Brain-damage--Patients--Biography. 4. Cancer--Patients--
    Biography. 5. Medical errors. I. Title.
    RA1056.5.H57 1997
    362. 1 ' 97481 ' 0092--dc21
    [B]   97-17592
                                                              CIP

DEDICATION

To Robin

DISCLAIMER

In Search of My Husband's Mind is a true story. The names of the author, her family, close friends, and some geographic locations are unchanged. The names of the hospitals and doctors have been changed. All other characters have been given pseudonyms or no names at all. Some geographic locations have also been changed.

CONTENTS

ACKNOWLEDGMENTS

I am deeply indebted to the good people who have read, checked, offered suggestions and encouraged my efforts with *In Search of My Husband's Mind.* I cannot single them out because the list is long and I would surely omit someone.

I do, however, have special thanks for Jim Churchill who found value in my first draft; for the late Bill Ryan, who persuaded author Anne Lamott to read the next draft; and to the latter because she shared her skills with me, showing me ways to narrow the focus of my story.

Finally, I thank Polly Bee. It was she who introduced me to Eugene Wheeler and the staff of Pathfinder Publishing. Their editorial suggestions have been thoughtful and mercifully infrequent.

PREFACE

In Search of My Husband's Mind is Winnie Hirsch's remembrance of medical care in a close personal relationship. Winnie writes evocatively and lovingly of the years she spent with her husband, Monroe Hirsch, an eminent optometrist who became the Dean of the School of Optometry at the University of California, Berkeley, and who eventually died of metastatic cancer. She wrote the story of his care and their relationship to bring to medicine a different vision of what ought to constitute good medical care, and to bring one more argument against the standard way in which physicians and hospitals deal with patients. She describes how the medical care Dr. Hirsch received over the several years before his death damaged their relationship and failed basic tests of quality and humanity.

Winnie writes in the context of the mystery of what went wrong in Monroe Hirsch's medical care, what mistakes were made, and what information was withheld from her. She discovers that Monroe's medical care was deeply flawed at times, but anyone who deals with medical care frequently will find her discoveries familiar. Medical care is rarely organized centrally in any manner, much less organized to deliver humane and quality care. The recent intrusion of the "health maintenance" concept and health maintenance organizations (HMO's) into the delivery of medical care has made no difference in this regard because the HMO concept is about controlling costs and making money, not improving the quality of care or delivering it in a more humane way.

The expectation that at least some one who is a professional in the medical care system will care about us, care about us in the sense that a loved one or friend will care, runs deeply. This compounds our disappointments when medical care lets us down. Her experience is ironic in this regard, because her husband was a medical professional, a professional at the highest level of his profession, and she worked closely with him throughout their relationship. Yet she expected medical professionals to care about her and her husband in a way that they are neither ready nor trained to provide.

She comes to realize, albeit too late to prevent her own medical tragedy, that quality, humane medical care can be insured only by patients themselves and by their loved ones and advocates. Reciting the rights of patients from "Patients Rights and Resources," she urges patients and their advocates to be assertive and informed, to monitor care, and to clearly speak out for the best interests of the patient.

Patients, family members, medical practitioners and administrators can gain much from reading this book.

Martin Gipson, Ph.D.
Head, Department of Psychology
University of the Pacific
Author, *Managing YOUR Health Care*

INTRODUCTION

This room, this tiny room, it is the place to which I could retreat when cries from a sick husband pushed me to the breaking point.

It is the place that could withstand my screams and the pounding of my fists when there was no one who could lessen my despair. It is the room to which I brought the necessities that kept me sane: my easy chair, our photographs and writings, the reminders of the love between Monroe and me.

These records are my memories. They show more happiness than evil; but it was a malevolence that attacked our happiness. It drove me night after night into transmitting my despair to paper and describing my frustrations and my sorrows.

Then, as my writings began to form into a tale, I was thrust beyond catharsis—into searching hospital and other records, into challenging the medical procedures that Monroe endured.

I had not thought of myself as a detective but that, in the end, was what I was driven to be; and this is my personal account, an exposé, if you will, of the negligence and transgressions I uncovered while trying so desperately to learn what had happened to the mind of the man I loved.

Winnie Hirsch
June 2, 1997

1

Monroe's leg was amputated February 3, 1978. He was quiet, sad, sedated when he told me he would lose his leg. In my own mind I thought he would be better off without the wasted limb because it had restricted his movement more than it had helped it. But only the one who loses a body part can feel the value of it.

On the morning after the amputation Monroe directed his gaze to the stump and asked, "When are they going to remove my leg?" Two days later he asked a physical therapist what had happened to it.

Eight or nine days later I came out of the elevator and found Monroe standing in the corridor in his bathrobe. I was shocked to see the full weight of his body hanging from his armpits as they pressed into the crosspieces of his crutches. His single leg provided balance rather than support. That was not the way a therapist had taught him to use crutches, and Monroe had a Ph.D. in physiology. He should have known that was not the way to use them.

Monroe seemed unable or unwilling to move. He stared, disheveled and disoriented, down the long corridor. It was as if he had no knowledge of where he was or what he was doing.

"So what's the matter with you?" a nurse joked, not waiting for an answer.

"I'm an old man," Monroe replied.

As the nurse passed by, she studied him quickly but quizzically, then continued her rounds.

The nurse's question sounded my worry. Something seemed wrong.

Something seemed seriously wrong with Monroe.

Ten days after the amputation I watched Monroe being taught the use of crutches on hospital stairs. He would need to negotiate stairs both at home and at work.

For a man as quick and as agile as Monroe had been, his progress on stairs seemed slow, but I thought he was afraid of falling. I thought he was too frightened to try. It scared me to look down the long flights of stairs the therapist had him practicing on, let alone try to go down the top flight on crutches. If the idea terrified me, what must it do to Monroe whose last fall led to his losing his leg?

I had read that an amputation often causes severe mental disturbances, so I asked for help.

A psychiatric consultant from the hospital came to talk to me. If he made a diagnosis of Monroe's problem, he didn't tell me. He did say I must be kind to Monroe, which seemed ridiculous at the time. How could I be other than kind to the man who had sustained my spirits for so many years?

Twelve days after the amputation I went to the nurses' station to express my concerns about caring for Monroe at home. Monroe's lethargy and lack of enthusiasm were two worries. Negotiating stairs was another. But my immediate and urgent concern was the correct way to bind the little that was left of Monroe's leg. I had been given one demonstration only by a member of the rehabilitation department, and he had considerable difficulty wrapping it because, he said, the stump was so short. I had never had the opportunity to take an Ace bandage in my hands and fix it firmly in position while not in any way constricting the circulation of blood in the stump. I was told never to do that. Monroe's doctor had cautioned me that if I did not bind it perfectly, Monroe might never be able to wear an artificial leg. With a warning like that, why had they never trained me?

At the nurses' station I stated emphatically that Monroe must not be discharged until the problems of stump-binding and stair-walking had been solved. Then, because nursing chores would soon tie me to Monroe's side, I took advantage of the free time remaining to me and went to a matinee.

When I returned I found Monroe dressed, packed and eager to go home. A discharge had gone through.

If I had been disemboweled, I would have felt happier than I did at having to drive almost two hours that night to our summer home in Ojai. Once there, it would be up to me to help a six-foot-tall new amputee into the house and into his bed. I was strong for my sixty years, but was I that strong? I was already unnerved at the prospect of binding an amputated leg without practicing the technique. And I also suspected Monroe had persuaded the doctor to let him go home— that he had told the physician that I was quite capable of taking care of him. Monroe had always, I fretted to myself, given me too much credit for competence.

I was too naive to know that I could have refused to take Monroe home even if the physician abandoned his responsibility. The hospital would have taken over. I have since found out that few patients are aware of this protection.

The discharge made me angry, frightened, discouraged. I have always been a bad sport about inconsiderate changes of plans and about being thrust into battle without armor. Traffic on the freeway did nothing to improve my disposition. I was so upset I didn't dare speak. My jaws hurt from keeping them locked together. I knew Monroe had suffered a grievous loss, and I was determined to not let the rage inside me erupt.

By the time we arrived home, I was tired, hungry and still angry. I parked the car in front of our porch, opened the house door, helped Monroe from the car and handed him his crutches. He placed them under his arms, hesitated, and said, "I don't know how to get up the step."

"You talked your way out of the hospital!" I exploded with uncontrolled fury, "You damn well better remember how to get up that step!" The intensity of my rage must have struck its mark for, in one continuous motion, he propelled himself over the step and through the door and into the house.

The speed and precision of his movement was so funny that my frenzy vanished. My cry of rage had not been kind, I warned myself. In the future I must be kinder, but for the time being, I was comforted by the ease with which he moved.

I didn't know it at the time, but Monroe and I were embarking on a new life. I would continue to love Monroe even in the face of frustrating and peculiar responses which were nothing like the responses of the man I married. We would continue to dwell under the same roof, but we would no longer live together as companions or as man and wife. We would no longer live our lives as we had lived them for so many years.

2

Six years before his amputation, Monroe had become Dean of the School of Optometry at the University of California in Berkeley. From our cottage in the hills we could see the pinnacled structures of San Francisco rise above the mist across the bay, and we could see the towering bell clock on the campus below us.

The University and Berkeley meant a lot to us. We felt at home there even though we had lived happily in southern California before moving north. We had met in Berkeley when we were students. We had dined in the same student restaurant frequently but had paid little notice of each other. He first held my attention when our paths crossed on the Berkeley campus. As he approached I noticed his long, thin face, serious beneath tousled, dark hair. A white collar peeped neatly above his navy sweatshirt. He appeared lost in thought, but suddenly the long, deep lines about his mouth lifted into a gentle smile. I smiled, too, not only because his expression was appealing but because his trousers, a rakish check of blue, black, and red, were outlandish and out of keeping with the seriousness of his face. Later, he told me that before leaving his home in New York, a salesman had convinced him they were "just the thing" for a campus in the wild west. He had already learned differently but had no money to replace his garish trousers.

A few days after that, while rounding a corner, we almost bumped into each other. This time he walked me home, but he was midway through a sentence when we reached my rooming house, so we kept on walking. He was so enthusiastic and expressed himself so vitally and logically that I became captivated by his ideas. I must have been starved for such intellectual companionship. I thought our relationship would be nothing more than that because he told me immediately about his girlfriend in New York. I remember feeling relieved that he was more or less engaged. It left me free to speak as I wanted to, and it meant I didn't have to be a coquette. I knew I was a failure as a flirt, and Monroe didn't seem to expect it of me. It was wonderful to feel relaxed and, a rarity for me, not at all self-conscious.

After that first encounter we met almost every evening for coffee and a walk. In those days, "roamin' in the gloamin'" was a popular activity for students without a car or money. Monroe had neither, but he always had something worth saying.

Then, as the semester drew to an end and it was time for Monroe to return to New York for the summer vacation, I knew I was in love with Monroe and he was attracted to me. I was also aware that he wasn't the sort of man who could have two sweethearts at the same time and not feel guilty about it. I didn't realize how guilty he felt until years later when I came across some reflections he had typed regarding his dilemma.

"My plight," he related, "was a source of amusement to my roommates. They began posting odds on which of the two women would get me as a husband... Gradually this became nerve-racking, and I became more and more convinced that something was wrong with me."

"I finally decided to be very scientific about the whole thing. I would list the faults and good points of each of my girlfriends, and choose accordingly . . ."

About the New York girl Monroe wrote: "Short, brunette, average appearance. We both like athletics and want to raise a family. Her disposition is perfect. She never says a harsh word. She's close to her mother and will never leave New York. Reads to excess. Jewish and a Democrat, 'same as myself'."

About me Monroe wrote: "Tall, blonde, better than average in appearance. She hates athletics and lives alone and likes it. Two quarrels thus far, but Irving (roommate) says she would follow me to China if I asked her. Reads to excess. A Gentile and a Republican."

Monroe sounded much less concerned about the differences in our religious background than about my conservatism. Before the end of the college year he had chalked up two more spats against me. "She maintained," Monroe wrote, "that she was going to be a career woman and, worse than that, she was going to remain a Republican. In fact she intimated that she didn't particularly care to get married..."

But love has a way of sorting things out. Four months after his mother died, Monroe asked me to marry him. It was shortly before graduation, and I didn't hesitate because my parents were soon to arrive in Berkeley. I knew my mother would throw a tizzy about my marrying someone without money, a Jew whose social background was not, in her opinion, as proper as hers. I had no intention of letting my mother's emotional outbursts drive Monroe back to the New York girl. I did not worry about my father's reaction. His brain was stronger than any prejudices he might have been brought up with.

We eloped the weekend before final exams.

Our first home was a three-room shanty which we leased for twenty dollars a month. In Berkeley that was a bargain even during the Depression. In addition, the first three months were free in exchange for painting the house. The "three months' free" had clinched the lease, for we had no money. Monroe would not officially be an optometrist until August when the results of the state board examinations were released. In the meantime, he was a gardener, and I was a typist at ten cents a page. Between times we painted the house.

On a day when Monroe and I were on stepladders and spattered with paint, my mother and father arrived in their new Hudson. My father emerged from the driver's seat and helped my mother through the door of the car. She placed her gloved hand over his arm and approached the house with angry face beneath a perfect crown of red-gold hair.

Monroe got down from his ladder. The two narrow-chested men peered at each other through myopic lenses. Then, just as my father extended a hand of kinship, my mother exploded, "Why couldn't you have waited for a church wedding?"

When I replied that it wouldn't have been kosher, my father turned away, grinning.

"Oh," fumed my mother, "You're laughing when you ought to be scolding her for running off with some... with some person... before..."

"Ee, Maud, stop your mithering," my father soothed in the Lancashire dialect of his youth. "There's nowt tha can do abat it now!" With that he went off for a walk with Monroe and left me alone to cope with my mother.

The next day my father got me aside and said, "Don't worry about your mother. She'll get used to his being a Jew.

But neither your mother nor I can understand how you managed to find such a poor one."

3

Thirty-six years later, in the spring of 1976, when Monroe was Dean of the School of Optometry, I noticed a lump on his right upper leg while he was dressing in our Berkeley house. I asked what it was, and he replied with genuine cheer, "It's a herniated muscle. I've been to a physician."

With that assurance, I forgot the lump but noticed it a few weeks later. "I don't care what that doctor said," I cried, "That thing's growing!"

He responded that he would see to it right after he conducted the upcoming graduation ceremonies. This time his voice was testy and worried.

A June biopsy revealed that the lump in Monroe's leg was not a hernia. It was cancerous, a spindle-cell sarcoma.

For many years an accepted approach to fighting cancer with any likelihood of success was immediate surgery following early detection and diagnosis. While early diagnosis remains important, techniques of treating cancers vary and are changing continually. Surgery is sometimes delayed and not done immediately.

In Monroe's case, he had detected the lump early, but the accurate diagnosis was not made until his cancer had plenty of time to grow.

After the graduation exercises Monroe consulted a highly recommended group of tumor specialists. These oncologists were connected with a university hospital in southern California. They decided to postpone surgery in the hope that most of the cancer cells could first be destroyed by chemotherapy. This would reduce the size of the tumor itself.

To begin with, a chemical called Adriamycin would be fed directly into the artery that supplied the cancerous muscle in Monroe's leg. By this method the cancer cells in the leg would receive the direct thrust of the killing chemical. Then, as it continued through Monroe's blood, it could be expected to destroy sarcoma cells if they split from the parent cancer.

For these pre-operative treatments, Monroe entered the hospital July 15, 1976, and was assigned to a private room. A cot was provided so that I could stay with him at night.

Monroe received the prescribed Adriamycin, suffering slight nausea only.

After a day of rest, the same procedure was to be followed, this time with a high dose of another cancer-killing chemical called Methotrexate. Before the Methotrexate was administered, the head of the oncology group stood at the foot of Monroe's bed and intoned that treatment of cancer by chemicals is based on the theory that the chemicals introduced into the body will first destroy the weaker cells. Cancer, stomach, and hair follicle cells are among the weaker ones, so the side effects of stomach distress and loss of hair can be expected. Before life-supporting cells are affected, the doctor went on, the killer chemicals are discontinued and the blood cleansed of them.

Monroe, under medication, smiled woozily and happily through the explanation. I, who was not medicated, felt the blood drain from my head. It was probable that Monroe would live through the chemical intake; but if the dosage was not terminated soon enough, his life-sustaining cells could die and Monroe could die in the process.

The head surgeon went on to say that Monroe would be the first patient on the west coast to receive Methotrexate so soon after Adriamycin. He said it had been done successfully in Boston on young people.

Extraordinary heroic measures, apparently, were being called upon to attack it.

I felt sick.

Over the next hours I watched Monroe's body move from a state of life to a state approaching death and then move slowly back to life. But the return seemed incomplete. Ten days after the chemotherapy session, Monroe was still lying abed most of the day in our summer house in Ojai. He didn't complain, but he seemed too weak and he talked too little. I became so worried I drove to a friend's house. I wanted to talk to her about Monroe; but the closer I got to her house, the sillier I felt about dumping my anxieties on her. I decided I had been worrying without cause and returned home.

Shortly thereafter, the phone rang and Monroe got up to answer it. A colleague wanted to know if we were going to the optometric camp out. Monroe said that we wouldn't miss it for the world. He hung up the receiver and retreated to his bed; but for a few moments he had responded so positively and happily that my anxieties dissolved into air.

I was not surprised that news of the camp out had stimulated Monroe's interest and enthusiasm. He had been one of the originators of the professional meeting in which lectures and discussions were held in campgrounds under an open sky. The youngest practitioners and their wives brought their babies and tents. The middle-aged campers brought their juveniles and recreational vehicles. The old or ill took cabins with hot running water.

We booked a room with running water.

So it was that a few days after the phone call we went to the camp out. Monroe stayed in the cabin bed much of the time, but he did get up for brief periods to fraternize with his cronies. It was a happy interlude before Monroe would have to return to the hospital for more chemotherapy.

The procedures that had been used on Monroe in July by the oncology group had brought marked destruction to the cancer cells. We were elated to see that the tumor was much smaller, and because of this success, the doctors wanted to do the same thing again. After that, Monroe would be given ten treatments by radiation. Without question, the doctors were trying to kill as many cancer cells as possible inside the tumor before surgery. In this way they hoped to reduce the opportunity for cancer cells to spread to other parts of the body.

The second round of chemotherapy and the radiation treatments passed uneventfully. September 14 was the date set for surgery. It would take place in the morning.

4

I caught a glimpse of Monroe's gray and shrunken face as the attendants wheeled his gurney toward the operating room. His once luxuriant hair was almost gone, the result of chemotherapy. Then they took him through the double doors beyond which I could not pass.

Surgery took over five hours, but I waited with wondrous serenity. I had wakened before dawn from a dream in which Monroe and I were sleeping side by side. In my dream I saw the cancerous lump billow slowly and gracefully out of his leg and into mine. I woke with an almost palpable calm around me.

Later, when the surgeon reported to me that the operation appeared a success, I was not surprised. He said that the chemotherapy had rendered the sarcoma inactive, that it seemed to have been limited to the large muscle at the front of the thigh, that it had not reached the bone. It had been a long operation because he had wanted to avoid blood transfusions and he also wanted to leave as much functional leg as possible. I thanked the surgeon.

I knew that when Monroe regained consciousness he would be more than pleased. He had been prepared to lose his whole leg if necessary, but the surgeon told me that a brace would be all that was needed to protect the damaged leg, and perhaps a cane.

Traume sind Schaume. I should have remembered that "dreams are but foam."

After discharge from the hospital, Monroe continued to recover his strength in our Ojai house. We slept together again in our king-sized bed, a pillow between us to protect his mending leg. I had placed our bed in the little room close to the kitchen because it was within calling distance of most of the house. The bed was so large and the room so small that only the narrowest of corridors separated one wall of the room from the foot of the bed. It looked ridiculous but proved convenient.

By October Monroe was still frail but getting around with his walker. His wound seemed to be healing except for an inch or so in the mid-section. On October 7 my throat hurt, so I went to sleep that night in the front bedroom to reduce Monroe's chance of getting a sore throat from me.

From a sound sleep I heard him lift and place his walker, step following step. Then I heard clang of metal and a heavy thud, and I was out of bed like a shot. I knew Monroe had fallen.

I found him on his back at the foot of the bed. Metal staples that had held the flesh together over the incision hung loose and twisted. The radiation-weakened tissue had not held. From more than twelve inches of his torn-apart wound, milk-colored matter was oozing. I hoisted him, dazed, onto the foot of the bed and frantically phoned the physician assigned to Monroe's recovery. Tarns, as the doctor shall be called, sounded more asleep than awake. He asked how much the wound had opened. I told him two inches, and I think I also said "wide." But he either failed to hear me in his state of half sleep or misinterpreted the meaning of "wide." Later he would tell me he thought the opening was two inches long, not that there was a two inch gap from one side of the wound to the other.

I had phoned Tarns because I thought Monroe should be taken to the hospital right away, but Tarns said, "No, have your family doctor pull the wound together and come in at our regular time."

Our family physician rushed to the house when I phoned him. He looked uncomfortable when I told him what Tarns had said, but he pulled the wound together without comment and bound it as the specialist had ordered.

Dr. Tarns may not have recalled my phone call, for he didn't telephone me the next day; nor did I call him, although I worried about it. Probably none of us, in the middle of the night, more asleep than awake, was competent to act with wisdom; but I, who could not help but be reminded the next day of what had happened, should have recognized that Tarns had not sensed the proportions of the damage. I have often thought that things might have been different:

if I had had more understanding of infection;
if I had been told what to look for;
if I had been less trusting of health care practitioners;
if I had learned to challenge physicians;
if I had learned to persist whenever I had doubts.

I should have moved immediately, but I did not. I should not have waited four days before driving Monroe to Tarn's office to show him the discouraging and unsightly wound.

The drive to that scheduled visit began before daybreak. I tried to be cheerful but couldn't. Monroe said little. He was worried. He knew the wound was infected. He told me it must have been infected all along because the small section in the middle had never healed and the white matter at the time of the fall had oozed from the length of the wound's opening.

The pink-tinged clouds of sunrise failed to dispel my fear that death was once again a possibility.

5

Dr. Tarns told me in the waiting room that Monroe's wound was so seriously infected he would have to return to the hospital immediately. He hadn't understood from our phone conversation, he explained, the extent of the problem.

"For future reference," I replied, and I think my manner was friendly, "the doctors where I live know I don't call for help unless it's serious. If I call for help, they come a-running..."

"We can't come running for every patient," he snapped in annoyance.

He seemed not to have understood what I said. Why did he think I was asking for special privilege when I was trying to tell him that physicians who knew me also knew that I didn't make unreasonable demands? I wondered how he could be so defensive so easily, but at the time I had more urgent things to worry about. Or so I thought.

In the hospital Monroe's wound was eventually cleared of its infection. After that, a skin graft was applied. It started growth of healthy new cells, called granular tissue. Hopefully, this tissue would eventually grow across the bone and cover it. At the time, however, the crossing was by no means complete. Some four inches of thigh bone were visible, and we had been warned that granular tissue sometimes fails to cover exposed bone.

In spite of that worry, Monroe and I were so optimistic we decided to send a report to our friends as a Christmas greeting. We composed a letter explaining that Monroe's incision extended from his 'guggle to his zatch,' an expression we swiped from James Thurber. Then we rejoiced that "round-the-clock dressings during October and November, plus high-protein milk shakes, plus a skin graft promise a December 'healing'..." We also announced the birth of our second grandson and our intention to attend the July fireworks of 2076 because we'd had to miss the bicentennial celebrations of 1976.

Friends phoned their delight at our high spirits.

Before we left the hospital, nurses taught me to dress Monroe's wound and bind the dampened gauze in place. It was imperative to prevent the exposed bone from drying out and becoming brittle. Sterile gauze dipped in sterile saline solution had to be folded into the wound every four hours, which I did on schedule for the next fifteen months. Monroe was also provided with a brace to protect his weakened thigh against breaking when he stood up.

Tarns admonished me never to let Monroe put much weight on that leg. "If the leg breaks," he warned me with a wag of his finger, "it will have to be amputated!" It was a warning thrust upon me often in the months to come. If I made a mistake Monroe would be damaged, and it was up to me not to let it happen.

When Monroe was discharged from the hospital in November, we knew that his wound might never heal and that he would have to return to the hospital for twelve more rounds of chemotherapy. Despite that, we were both euphoric: Monroe would be home for Christmas, and he could get about with the help of a brace and a cane.

6

Many years before, soon after Monroe became a student of optometry at Berkeley, one of the toughest teachers in the department gave an examination. Monroe misspelled *lens* ten times. After each *lense*, the teacher put a minus ten, which left Monroe with a zero for his efforts. At the end of the test the teacher wrote, "I see you haven't learned to spell *lense* yet."

Monroe was furious about receiving a zero on an otherwise perfect paper, but he thought the professor's comment was funny. He began to pay attention to his spelling in addition to more important matters. Before long that same contentious teacher recognized in Monroe a bright and promising student and hired him as a helper.

The dean of the school at that time also noticed Monroe's growing skills and absorption in scientific principles. Following graduation he urged Monroe to continue his education and obtain a doctor of philosophy degree. Monroe demurred. He didn't have money to stay in school any longer.

Meanwhile, the United States had become embroiled in war against Germany and Japan. One day the dean collared Monroe and said that Stanford University needed an optometrist for a research project sponsored by the Air Force. Specifically, the Air Force wanted to know the least light that could be used on a carrier deck and still permit planes to land safely. The less illumination that could be used, the less vulnerable the carrier would be to an enemy.

Monroe was told that if he took the job, it would allow him to work for a higher degree while earning a research stipend. But I was pregnant and Monroe hesitated. With years of financial insecurity in his past, he was very concerned about making a living. I, on the other hand, had no experience with poverty, so I had no fear of it. Consequently, I opted for Stanford University immediately.

We moved there in 1943. Jeff, our only child, was born in November of that year.

During the war years, Stanford University was a hive of activity. Quick solutions were often needed to save or protect life on a large scale; but during the time we were at Stanford, I never saw the need for speed interfere with careful scientific investigation. The need for getting on with a task, however, led many professors and research workers to improvise and build their own equipment rather than await delivery from the back-logged building department. Morale was high; ingenuity was higher; and it was understood that anyone so careless as to leave boards or nails around could expect to see them next day built into someone else's equipment.

Monroe took to building his own equipment as eagerly as a raccoon takes to garbage cans. He had always liked rough carpentry, saying it got rid of his aggressions: that pounding on nails was better than pounding on people.

He was assigned a long section of basement beneath the physiology building in which to construct his equipment and perform his experiments. In these windowless 'catacombs,' the amount of lighting could be controlled carefully.

The first need of Monroe and others in the vision laboratory was to find people who could judge distance accurately. This was necessary because they would be participating in experiments as if they were pilots. Consequently, the testing equipment would look like that used in selecting pilots, but it would be much larger.

First, two parallel rails were run the length of the corridor. Then, an upright rod was mounted on each rail. These rods were identical. Anyone looking through a slit into the corridor could see the two rods, but not the rails or anything else. As the rods were moved toward or away from an observer, he had to signal when they passed each other. It seems easy, but many people signal when the rods are far apart. Ability to judge depth accurately may not seem important, but it's important if a person is parking a car; and it's very important if a pilot is landing a plane.

Not long before the war in Europe ended, Monroe came home and announced that he'd never be able to say he'd won the war. The Air Force, he said, had found a safe way to land planes at night: crews wearing fluorescent suits were guiding pilots safely onto totally dark carrier decks. No illumination was needed.

Nonetheless, Monroe's research in the vision laboratory was basic and important. Over a period of five years, he and his colleagues not only researched how the amount of light affects judgment of depth, but how judgment is altered if other clues are involved. For example, If one rod is bigger than another, the bigger rod may appear closer even though they are the same distance away.

During this period, Monroe was studying for a Ph.D. and working in the optometric clinic at the University of California. He was exhausting himself, but in spite of all his efforts, we were falling behind in our bills. I was busy with baby Jeff, and my thesis typing brought in little cash. One month we were greatly relieved to find that there was still forty-six cents left in our checking account.

My expectations for our Christmas/Chanukah celebration were bleak; but if Monroe was dismayed, he didn't show it. Instead, he converted Jeff's baby stroller into a "locomotive" and built me a stand for holding the big dictionary he had given me the previous year.

When my parents arrived for the holidays, my non-mechanical father was overwhelmed by the ingenuity of his son-in-law. "You have a very satisfactory husband," my father told me, "and a very satisfactory child." That was praise indeed from my very reserved father.

Later that day Dad gave Monroe a check big enough to cover a year's rent. "A whole year's rent!" Monroe and I whispered to each other, overjoyed that we would have a roof over our head and meat on the table in the months ahead.

Monroe received his doctorate in philosophy from Stanford University's School of Medicine in 1947. Too poor to afford a cap and gown, he watched the proceedings from the audience.

The following summer, the vertebrae in my neck were dislocated during an automobile accident en route to Salt Lake City. Following traction, my neck had been put in a brace, a standard procedure in those days. I remained for a month under medical care in Salt Lake City. (This was not standard practice. The osteologist thought I had been discharged.) By the time members of the Stanford physiology department saw me, the brace had rubbed sores into my shoulders and under my chin. In addition, my neck had been fixed in a brace so long I could no longer hold my head erect or turn it. I had been told I would wear the brace the rest of my life.

The Stanford physiologists, M.D.s and Ph.D.s, held a seminar to discuss my problem. Pooling their varied skills and up-to-date knowledge, they defeated the sores in short order. They offered ideas to tone my neck and shoulder muscles to free me from the brace.

The skill with which these scientists, by integrating their knowledge, rid me of my problems gave me a firm conviction that a university medical school was the place to go if a complicated health problem was involved. That was the reason why, many years later, when Monroe elected to have his cancer taken care of by a similar university group, I felt great confidence in his choice.

In the year of my accident, Stanford promoted Monroe to acting assistant professor of physiology. But even with this promotion, Monroe's salary was low and prices had continued to rise after the war. That was why the three of us in 1949 climbed into our battered car and headed for southern California. There, at double his Stanford salary, Monroe became an associate professor at the Los Angeles College of Optometry, then located adjacent to the University of Southern California.

7

Years later at the end of 1977, Monroe was scheduled to receive additional chemotherapy as a follow-up to the surgical removal of the cancer in his leg. The purpose was to ward off the return of cancer. Each round of therapy would be given four or five weeks apart in the hospital, each treatment taking about three days.

Such chemotherapy was based on the assumption that cells from the removed cancer could have split off before surgery and might still be present and reproducing somewhere in the body. For such chemical treatments to have an opportunity to succeed, they must be given at regular intervals and started soon after surgery. If not, lurking cancer cells might reproduce and gain the upper hand. But if everything went as hoped, no escaped cancer cell would survive beyond the last treatment.

After each Methotrexate treatment, an antidote would be administered at frequent and exact intervals in the hospital and continued at home. Again, I was admonished that the antidote had to be given to Monroe on time at home, exactly as directed, or he could die.

While the timing of the chemotherapy was necessary to fight the cancer cells, it was unfortunate that it had to come so soon after the infection in the incision in Monroe's leg had been eradicated. It was unfortunate because with each chemotherapy treatment, many newly formed granular tissue cells which had started to cross the exposed thigh bone would be destroyed along with remaining, undesirable cancer cells. Between sessions, granular tissue would be produced, but with each treatment, some of the new growth would be lost. Nevertheless, when we changed the dressing between sessions, we could see that the granular tissue was gaining. We held high hopes that the tissue would cross the bone so the wound could heal.

Except for patients whose treatment called for isolation, there were no private rooms in the cancer ward. Each room accommodated two patients who were either recovering from surgery or receiving chemotherapy.

The most irascible of Monroe's roommates was a Nevada rancher who was paying directly for hospital care because he was not insured. One day, shortly before the nurses changed shift, he had to be helped to his commode. The nurse reminded him that he must not get up without help under any circumstances. Then she left her shift, forgetting to relay his predicament to the incoming nurse. Forty-five minutes later the rancher rose in Olympian rage from his latrine. He dressed. With his walker clanging before him, he stormed out of the hospital, cursing as he went.

At the time I thought it was funny. Later I have wondered why I didn't have his courage. For whatever fate he eventually suffered, it couldn't have been worse than Monroe's.

A young car salesman was Monroe's fifth roommate. He was recovering from the removal of a cancerous tumor on his arm. He and his wife wept for joy when they heard the operation was a success. Later I heard him tell his wife how Monroe's jokes made him laugh.

By July Monroe was halfway through his treatments. All had appeared to go well. Between treatments Monroe saw a few patients, helped raise funds for the new wing of the optometry school in Berkeley and awarded degrees during its 1977 commencement exercises. Our son went to the exercises to photograph Monroe. I asked him to protect Monroe as well. I asked Jeff to see that no children run into him or that some backslapper not force him to put his weight on his bad leg. "He'll do all right if he can see what's coming," I said. "The main thing is to guard the rear."

Later Jeff wrote:

When my father finished giving out all the diplomas and the ceremony concluded, I stayed talking with my father and his friends so we'd be the last ones out of the crush of the crowd. Instead, he pointed to the far side of the crowd as the place he wanted to go, and off he went with his cane, ever his own man, happily plunging right into the thick of the crowd, talking with people, pumping flesh....

8

Following Monroe's August chemotherapy in 1977, he was not allowed to leave the hospital at the expected time. He had to remain an extra day to receive more antidote because, we were told, too much Methotrexate remained in his blood.

He was released at the end of the fourth day, in time for us to attend the optometric camp out in Big Sur. As soon as we got there, I changed Monroe's bandages. When I pulled off the old gauze, a multitude of fire-colored "bubbles," infinitesimally small, seethed and wormed inside the wound and did not subside for several hours. When they did, the granulated tissue had disintegrated with a thoroughness that had never occurred before. Frightened at the damage I had seen and fearing what might be happening elsewhere in his body, I telephoned the oncology group and reached their liaison nurse. She assured me that granular tissue always recedes after Methotrexate and that what was happening should be expected. I insisted that this was different, that we could see things happening that hadn't happened before. She repeated her statement with no hint of concern. Her assurances left me greatly relieved.

On our third day at Big Sur, Monroe became querulous and demanding. By the fourth day he had quieted.

A month later we went to Berkeley to attend the official "kick-off" of the campaign to raise money to furnish the new wing of the optometry school. A professional fund raiser had written prepared statements for each speaker on the dais. His purpose was to avoid duplication of subject matter and guarantee brevity. Monroe approved these goals but disapproved of parroting another person's words; so he delivered his speech in the time allotted on the appropriate topic, but in his own words which were more pertinent than the prepared text.

I was proud of his competence and integrity.

When Monroe returned to Los Angeles for his September chemotherapy, I was still worried about the ugly activity in Monroe's wound during the camp out. I mentioned it to a nurse who was in Monroe's room. "Oh," she exclaimed, "that must have been the bad batch of Methotrexate!"

I shall probably never find out whether the Methotrexate was bad or whether the nurse was misinformed, but of this I am sure: Monroe and I never again saw an advance of granular tissue inside Monroe's wound although we looked for it hopefully and fearfully every four hours for the next few months at every change of dressing.

During Monroe's October chemotherapy treatment, I was in his room when a temporary replacement for Dr. Tarns appeared. He was instructing a group of medical students. As they surrounded Monroe's bed, the physician displayed Monroe's open wound, the thigh bone clearly visible thirteen months after surgery. The physician asked the students to observe how well the wound was healing.

"You've got a big imagination!" I blurted out in contradiction to the doctor's statement. I couldn't believe any teacher-physician would make such a misleading statement to students in his charge!

The doctor paused, then laughed a sharp laugh. The students joined with him. They left immediately without inquiring why I was so exasperated. I felt remorseful for saying what I did. Above all, I did not want my fears conveyed to Monroe. I had not meant to be rude to the physician, but I wanted the doctors to pay attention, to not gloss over evidence of a problem that was clearly visible. I wanted them to look the problem straight in the face—so we could face it, too.

I had already come to believe that Monroe's wound would never heal, that every day for the rest of his life Monroe's wound would be open and in need of sterile bandages to keep the exposed bone moist. No matter how I held my fright from Monroe, I knew that his leg was in jeopardy and that any undue activity could cause it to break. I believe Monroe knew this, too, although he never said so. With each chemotherapy after "the bad one," he seemed to withdraw. He seemed to be protecting himself against a fear he never expressed. He seemed to build a wall between himself and others.

Without ever stating that the wound might never heal and without arguing the alternatives, Dr. Tarns did offer a course of action: Monroe could spend much of the next two years in bed undergoing a deep graft to cover the wound, his legs immobilized and joined together.

With the possibility of a return of cancer lurking steadily in the background, and with the possibility that he might not live long enough for the graft to succeed, Monroe decided against the graft and risked the loss of his leg.

As it turned out, either decision was a bad one.

Across the years our friendship with Irving, Monroe's college roommate, never waned. Though we lived miles apart, we had long celebrated New Year's Eve with him and with Nora, his wife. During the holidays that followed Monroe's final chemotherapy in 1977, he was subdued as usual following the treatment, but he joined our chatter. We toasted Monroe's return to the university and the end of his chemotherapy.

That evening floats back to me as a happy memory.

Another evening, one month later, comes at me in jabs and spurts and broken pieces, never as a whole. I watch Monroe take his grandsons down the hallway of our Berkeley house and into their room to look at their toys. I see Monroe's hand on the corridor floor. I cannot see the rest of him. I run to the room. He is on his back struggling to get up, but his leg in its brace is not straight any more. It's not right. I know it's not right. I know it is broken and will be cut off.

I see Jeff race to the phone. Lights from the fire engine and ambulance flash in the street. Neighbors rush to the house. I pull chile rellenos from the oven before they burn, saying hysterically that Monroe's leg will be amputated because the doctor told me so and seeing terror in my daughter-in-law's face. She is gripping her babies to her breast because she thinks it is they who caused their grandfather to fall.

She did not know his femur was too fragile to sustain weight any longer. It fractured on its own, and that is why he fell.

An ambulance jet carried us south to the hospital. Dr. Tarns couldn't save his leg. The bone was too brittle, so the leg was cut off.

That was on February 3, 1978.

9

Thirty-one years earlier we lived in Los Angeles because of Monroe's job at the optometric school. Our stay in LA was brief. We missed the cultural amenities that Los Angeles lacked at the time, and we missed the compactness of Stanford and the liveliness of San Francisco.

Although we never opened our arms to Los Angeles, we thrived. We bought our first house and a beagle, and Monroe was soon promoted to full professor and director of research. Our years of penury were over.

Students said Monroe was the first to make them understand that optometry was more than a pair of eyeglasses; that optometrists must look at things scientifically and not accept a statement or instrument reading without making sure it agreed with other evidence.

He wrote a "scientific" spoof with many clues that it was a hoax. He put his name on it and gave it to students to analyze. They discussed it and most nodded agreement and didn't challenge it. Finally, one student volunteered that

Monroe's "theory" was hard to accept but, because Monroe's name was on it, it must be true.

That was too much for Monroe. "It's not the name you're supposed to examine!" he roared, "It's the evidence!"

Jeff, early in the 1950s, began to reason sequentially and in perfect imitation of Monroe. He would remove his newly acquired spectacles, contemplate them for a second, and proceed to punctuate each point of his reasoning with a forward jab of his glasses.

By that time I had given up any notions of a career and had become a Cub Scout den mother. In his spare time, Monroe was a den father and travelled extensively as a guest lecturer. He made so many trips to the state capitol to testify on optometric bills that he was known at the school as "Senator Hirsch."

Meanwhile, Monroe was growing restless at the Los Angeles college. Time allotted to research was rare and had to be cadged in spare moments or late at night. During his fourth year on the faculty, changes in the board of trustees produced an anti-intellectual majority in that body. One trustee explained that doctors of philosophy didn't need to get a pay raise because they weren't practical enough to compete in private practice.

Monroe took that statement as a personal challenge. He decided to find a good place to establish a private practice. He would no longer be restricted to cities where optometry was taught. As he later explained to a reporter, "The decision set us free... We had the whole country to choose from..."[1]

All we needed was a town we liked that was large enough to support a practice.

One spring day in 1953, after leaving a convention in Santa Barbara, and still thinking of a place for a private practice,

Monroe steered our car onto a two lane road that led through the Ventura oil fields and into a river valley lined with sycamores and oaks. The road topped a steep grade and entered a narrow valley of oak woodland and citrus groves surrounded by shrub-covered hills and jagged mountains. It was serene, inviting, spectacular.

"This is where I want to live!"

"Me too!" I replied to Monroe.

Then we came to a sign that read OJAI. As we drove past it, we saw that the population was less than two thousand. Not enough to support an optometrist, or so we thought, because the rule-of-thumb called for five thousand people. With dampened spirits we proceeded into the village itself.

Ojai's commercial district was only two blocks long in 1953, its architecture Spanish. El Roblar Hotel took up one square block, its front facing south. Across the street, the county library and a motion picture theater flanked three professional offices, two stores and an empty building.

The long block east of the hotel held a series of graceful arches that faced a park of rugged oaks and sycamores. Most of the town's stores slumbered behind the arches. On one corner of the park stood the post office with its Spanish bell tower.

Monroe parked his car to scout the town. He introduced himself to a passerby as an optometrist thinking of coming to Ojai. The response was immediate. Ojai needed an optometrist—if he would make his home here and didn't live in some other place like the optometrist who was here before. Monroe asked two others. They gave the same response.

We learned about Ojai's youth tennis tournament, art center, and music festival. I saw quality merchandise in the stores. Ojai was no ordinary small town. It was becoming irresistible. But the population was too small, we reminded ourselves, to make a living from optometry. Then we waved away that worry. Monroe could make extra money lecturing.

We looked for office space. There was only one building available, right next to the other professional offices across from the hotel. Its rent was so reasonable we almost leased it that day, but Monroe loved teaching. He had spent hard years training for it. To turn his back on a college career took courage. We retreated to Los Angeles to think it over. We did little else during the next week.

Monroe made further inquiries. He learned that there were more people in the surrounding valley than in the city of Ojai itself. "Also," Monroe observed, "I noticed a lot of older people here, and everyone past forty needs glasses. We can make a go of it in Ojai!"

We wasted no more time. We drove to Ojai the next weekend, rented the vacant building and hired a carpenter to remodel it. We returned jubilant, excited, and not a little scared, to Los Angeles.

Monroe left at the end of the school year to lecture in Canada. Jeff and I barely beat the moving van to Ojai. I worked with the carpenter on the office plans. By the time Monroe returned from his trip two weeks later, the partitions were up and the doors in place. Monroe was pleased with my efforts.

As we worked together to put the finishing touches on Monroe's office, local people dropped in to offer help or lend equipment. Before the flooring was down, Monroe examined his first Ojai patient. Others insisted on being examined before the practice was officially open.

"I should have written earlier," Monroe responded to a cousin shortly after returning from his Canadian lecture, "but I have so much mail to get out that I dictated to Winnie until 1:00 AM for 3 nights—and we sent out over 40 letters in that period. We have a lot of research stuff cooking and ...I got the job as Assistant Editor of the American Journal of Optometry and begin editing in September. How anyone who spells and punctuates the way I do got that job, I don't know."

The editing job gave Monroe a salary when he needed it. It also kept him in close touch with developments in research. Eventually, Monroe became its editor—and a good speller.

When word reached optometrists in the academic world that Monroe had left teaching for a practice in a town they had never heard of, they were shocked. It was a loss to education. In order that his research could be published under its name, the University of California's Optometry School took Monroe on as a consultant.

It wasn't until September that we had time to mail announcements of the opening of the office. Two days later our home phone rang. I answered and heard a jubilant Monroe, "You've got to help me! I'm getting so many calls I can't get anything done."

I hastened to the office to become Monroe's receptionist. I held the job for eleven years. People often remarked how well we got on together.

ENDNOTES

1 The Ventura County Star-Free Press, July 2, 1967.

10

Because Ojai was the sort of town where dogs sleep in the street and children run free, Jeff went exploring often. A favorite haunt was the post office where he studied the pictures of desperadoes wanted by the F.B.I. The woman behind the post office counter knew everyone in town. She decided that any parent of Jeff was worthy of support. She briefed us on the habits of a small town. She warned us against ten people who cheated whenever they could, but advised us not to question the credit of anyone else. If we asked about credit, she said, we would probably alienate the wealthiest and most influential people because they often looked like tramps in their overalls and frayed tennis shoes.

It was good advice. Monroe had one of the lowest losses in California throughout his years in practice. It is also true that I used applied sociology. I made sure that those who lived in one of the few transient areas of the valley made a down payment.

Once I overheard a patient tell Monroe, "I came for an examination because I heard your wife brag about you. Whenever a wife is that proud of her husband, he has to be good."

Before long we were looking for a house to buy. There were few available in those days, but I managed to find a small and artistic house built of redwood. It was only slightly beyond our means.

Just then my parents arrived for a vacation and to look over the town in which we had settled. I told dad I wanted to show him a special house. If he approved of it, I planned to ask him to lend us money to buy it. He liked the house but misjudged my intention in showing it to him. "It's just right," he said as he whipped out his checkbook, "I'll buy it for your mother!"

Foiled by my father's love for my mother, Monroe and I settled for second best, a house that was dark and drab and in need of repair, but one we could afford.

On the day we put it in escrow, the newspaper reported that the house had been raided by police and the front door kicked in. Monroe phoned the chief of police. "Please," Monroe urged, "take it easy on that house you raided last night. We just bought it."

"Glad you did," the chief retorted. "We've had trouble with that place. You just bought the whole red light district of Ojai."

One of Monroe's first patients was a woman in her thirties. Headaches oppressed her soon after she woke in the morning. No one had brought her relief.

Monroe determined that the difference in power between her two eyes was so extreme that no brain could tolerate it. Such an anomaly is rare. Few doctors know how to calculate the lenses that can comfort the sufferer. Only large institutions are likely to have the expensive equipment that can test it easily and accurately.

Monroe had the knowledge but not the equipment. In order to confirm his diagnosis, he resorted to a variation of the depth perception tests he had performed at Stanford. He held his arms horizontally in front of him and tilted his hands to a vertical position as if they were rods. He moved them back and forth slowly. He asked which hand appeared closer to her. Then he stood on a stool and did the same thing. Then he got down on his knees with his elbows on the floor and asked the same question.

At that moment I came into the refracting room to tell Monroe of an urgent call. He left to answer it. Not knowing that I was the doctor's wife, she beckoned me to her side and whispered, "Do you think that man has any idea about how to examine eyes?"

"He most certainly does!" I responded with all the confidence in the world. I had to be emphatic because it was obvious that no doctor had ever tested her eyes while crawling around on the floor.

Based upon lengthy mathematical calculations, Monroe ordered lenses for her. After they were fitted to her, she became comfortable for the first time in her life. She moved to another state, but returned year after year to see Monroe.

To find out how patients in a small town learned about Monroe, we put dots on a map to show where the patients lived. A dot would appear in one location and soon other dots would appear around the nucleus. In our minds we could see individuals talking over their fences; we could see the word pass from one street to the next. Before long, good things were being said about Monroe not only in Ojai but in nearby towns as well.

In all the time I worked with Monroe I never saw him take a patient into his consultation room without first studying past records on the patient. He did this to detect trends or deviations. He spent a long time talking with patients and listening to them. He picked up enough information during the consultation to uncover the probable cause of the patient's problem and to gauge the approximate lenses that would be needed if lenses were the solution. Sophisticated instruments, he said, could improve the precision of a prescription to solve a problem, but could never replace intelligent listening, observation, knowledge, and reasoning ability.

All health care practitioners should emboss that last thought onto their brains in flashing lights. All too many don't know, don't observe, don't listen, and don't reason.

11

Following the amputation of Monroe's leg early in 1978 I encouraged him to get back to work at the university. I thought such activity would give him less time to worry about the possible return of cancer or to grieve for the loss of his leg. I knew that the loss of a limb is one of the most traumatic events an individual can suffer, but I believed Monroe would compensate for his handicap. I thought he would put his inventive mind to work for himself as he had for others. I was sure he would rig our house with Rube Goldberg devices to satisfy his whims and make up for the lost leg.

That is why, after we returned to Berkeley, I expressed pleasure rather than annoyance at his method of getting up and down stairs. He had been instructed to negotiate stairs by tucking both crutches under the arm farthest from the banister before rising up or dropping down to the next step. In this way, one arm received support from the banister while the other arm received support from the doubled-up crutches. By moving in the proper way, Monroe would have both crutches with him when he reached the top or the bottom of the stairway.

Monroe, however, hit upon his own method: At the bottom of the stairs, he threw one crutch to the next landing; or, at the top, he threw one crutch down the stairs. His method was hard on the walls and hard on my nerves. I found myself expecting the sound of a falling body after the clatter of the falling crutch. Nonetheless, I decided that I must show pleasure that he was managing stairs without hesitation and that I must keep my nerves in harness.

A pair of old friends picked me up at the airport and commented on Monroe's agility, healthy appearance, and cheerfulness; but after we got home he seemed not to know what to say to them. He sat beside them, looked at them, seemed bewildered, and retreated across the room. He repeated this pattern several times, then went to bed.

Monroe could not yet drive, so I acted as his chauffeur to and from work. As a result, I was often at the School of Optometry. Sometimes I found Monroe asleep behind his desk in his private office. Often I heard his secretary beg him to prepare material so she could have it ready on schedule. I heard him put off such tasks with "tomorrow."

I could see that Monroe was neglecting jobs that had to be done. With each day I became more apprehensive that he would make an error or omission that would hurt the school.

He was often abrasive and inconsiderate to employees he had liked and who had done no wrong.

At home he said he wanted to quit work. Whenever I encouraged him to do so, he replied, "Tomorrow;" but on the morrow he didn't quit.

My thoughts were:
- Worry about job.
- Loss of a leg.
- Possible return of cancer.

- Classic causes for depression.

In addition, and shortly before he lost his leg, Monroe's father died, the last of his immediate family. Loss of a loved one.

Another reason to suspect depression.

It was logical to assume Monroe was depressed, and it was often suggested to me that he was. But whether he was or was not, I knew something was terribly wrong with him. He needed help for his mind.

On my own I went to a psychiatrist. I told him about Monroe's erratic behavior and the way he was handling his job. I related that a friendly colleague had observed to me, "He acts as if he's looking for a fix."

When I got home from the psychiatrist's office, I persuaded Monroe to go with me on my next visit.

Before that visit was over, the psychiatrist told Monroe to stop using Dalmane, the hypnotic agent Tarns had prescribed to help Monroe sleep. Some people, the psychiatrist stated, became disoriented by Dalmane. Monroe volunteered that he wanted to quit his job. The psychiatrist agreed that Monroe should enjoy life and stop working. The next day Monroe turned in the resignation I had written for him. He also stopped using Dalmane, and his behavior seemed less erratic. Or was I wishful thinking?

Monroe refused further psychiatric help.

When Monroe next saw Tarns, I detained him as he rushed to see another patient. I told him that the Dalmane he had prescribed had increased Monroe's mental problem and that it must never be given to him again.

12

In June of 1978 a crowd gathered for dinner to say fare-well to Monroe as Dean of the School of Optometry. He had prepared no speech and I assumed no speech was expected of him.

I was enjoying the brief and witty tributes being offered to Monroe when a speaker concluded by turning toward Monroe and praising him as "Mr. Optometry."

With that, Monroe stood up and began to speak. What he spoke made sense. At least, each section made sense, but there were too many sections and they did not coalesce into a whole. He spoke of his past aspirations and the achievements of optometry, but the precision and flair with which he had formerly made his points were absent. He rambled, and his ramblings continued. I felt desperate.

Screened by the tablecloth, I pinched his good leg. It was trembling with fatigue, but he went on. I pinched him again. Then, when he introduced the subject of optometry's relationship to socialized medicine, I pinched him hard.

Suddenly and without warning he announced, "I know I've talked too long because my wife just pinched me, but I don't know how to stop!" He sat down abruptly. Genuine laughter and applause followed. The crisis was over and the party went on to a merry end.

At the time I was terribly upset. It still upsets me, but when it leaps into my mind against my will, I also remember that when he spoke of the things he had done, he didn't say "I." He said "we."

That makes me cry.

It makes me cry in the English sense of "Have a good cry, lass. You'll feel better for it."

In 1953 when we moved to Ojai, Monroe didn't ramble. He was in command of himself. The world before him seemed without barriers.

He kept up his academic work and got into politics. He campaigned to have a city manager for Ojai and was elected to the city council in 1956. He sought to save the beauty of Ojai by careful use of land. He voted with the majority to preserve a magnificent stand of oak trees against a developer's bulldozer.

In 1958 Monroe was chosen to be mayor by his fellow council members and, for the first time, the city's ordinances were codified.

Years later a man passed me in an Ojai restaurant. Then he retraced his steps to say, "When your husband was on the city council, I went to council meetings for no other reason than to hear him talk. He always had the right word... so articulate..."

In those days Monroe worked by day at his office and by night in his study—unless he was attending a meeting. His energy rarely flagged.

His optometric practice grew, so we built a larger office in 1957. It was a half mile from our house and Monroe usually lunched at home. One day he arrived late, carrying a tray of raspberries and grinning broadly. He explained that the car of a ninety-year-old man who lived near us had broken down in front of the office. The old man had come into the office at noon to ask for a lift home. Monroe agreed.

Monroe had left his car unlocked. When he got to it he found it filled with boxes of raspberries, the gleanings of the old man's garden. Along the way, the man asked Monroe to detour first to one street, then to another, to complete his raspberry delivery route. By the time Monroe dropped the man at his own door, fifteen minutes remained of Monroe's lunch time. He had bought the remaining raspberries to avoid further detours.

About this time Monroe began a fifteen-year research project. Twelve hundred Ojai Valley boys and girls were involved at the start; each was five or six years old. By refracting these same students each year until they finished high school, Monroe would have a continuous pattern of their individual changes in near and farsightedness and in astigmatism.

At the start of the project we joked that we'd never live long enough to see its end. Three years later, after testing long lines of jostling students, we joked about letting the project die before it killed us. Fortunately, positive trends encouraged Monroe to continue. Before long, he found that children who were markedly farsighted when they started school tended to remain markedly farsighted. This contradicted a prevailing theory. Consequently, when it became clear through the work of Monroe and others that high degrees of farsightedness would not disappear as children grew older, it also became obvious that eyeglasses for farsightedness should be prescribed as soon as possible. By doing so, a farsighted child would not be handicapped in doing close work in school.

In spite of families moving out of the valley, Monroe obtained a continuous record on more than three hundred pairs of eyes by the end of the fifteen years. Approximately eighty percent of these children showed no change in their refractive state throughout their school life; but about twenty percent of those whose eyes were in the normal range as they started school did develop nearsightedness.

The development of nearsightedness during school years had, as Monroe explained to a reporter for the Ojai Valley News in 1973, "suggested to scientists as early as 1850 in Germany that school work caused nearsightedness. This is not true. Nearsightedness has to do with the size of the optical parts. If the parts continue to grow out of proportion, nearsightedness is brought about." If nearsightedness had been due to school work, almost all students would have changed. The study revealed, however, that the big majority did not change.[1]

ENDNOTE

1   The Ojai Longitudinal Study confirmed earlier research by Hirsch and Weymouth. Their work, done in the 1940s, was incorporated posthumously in 1991 as the first three chapters of *Refractive Anomalies: Research and Clinical Applications*, Edited by Theodore Grosvenor and Merton C. Flom; Butterworth-Heinemann, publishers.

13

Between 1960 and 1968 Monroe co-edited three text books. This was a period of our lives when our library seemed always stuffed with pages to be proofread and corrected.

In 1965 Jeff moved out of our orbit into the Peace Corps and a life of his own. Shortly before this, Mike and Robin drove into Ojai and into our lives. As a new graduate in optometry, Mike came to Ojai to discuss working with Monroe.

Mike had been such an outstanding student that it was almost assured he would be an acceptable partner for Monroe. But in a small town in those days, a doctor's wife came under close scrutiny. Before committing ourselves to Mike, we wanted to see if Robin would fit into the community.

She turned out to be nice looking, pleasant, quiet, but disappointingly unintellectual. Nonetheless, we overlooked any flaws in Robin because Monroe was so pleased with Mike. We met socially from time to time after Mike was hired. I enjoyed these events because of the compatibility between Mike and Monroe rather than for any feeling I had for Robin.

At the time I was unaware that she was beginning to stir from her cocoon, that she would soon display a deep awareness of the world around her. "But it wouldn't have happened without Monroe," she told me some time later. "As he talked and told stories of his childhood, I could feel his thoughts just as if he were standing at a tenement window in New York. He saw society not from the safety of a San Diego suburb as I did, and not from a Utah mountain top as you did, but from a tenement with no security except from the love and compassion within it. His view was clear; he knew every facet of a city; the causes and complexities of social injustice; and he could empathize with the underdog.

"He was one of the few people in my life who didn't think the losers in this world get exactly what they deserve! He guided me, not by always accepting my choices, but by understanding them."

Monroe, she said, increased her sense of community. Before long she embraced the ecology movement and committed herself to recycling waste. She cooked with a solar oven, rotating it often to catch the maximum rays of the sun. She learned the workings of solar water heating so thoroughly that she and her friends convinced the school board to install a solar heater on top of its cafeteria. Then she rounded up volunteers to get the solar heating installed at no cost to the school.

Probably without being aware of it, she changed in a few short years from a pleasantly pretty girl to a woman of rare grace and beauty. She had a knack of materializing whenever help was needed.

In time she became my anchor to sanity.

14

Following his retirement from the university in 1978, I returned with Monroe to Ojai and felt an overpowering sense of relief. I was tired from packing and closing the Berkeley house. I was tense from worry about Monroe's unexpected, obdurate and confusing behavior and looked forward to the quiet of Ojai where we could "sort things out."

I felt sure Monroe would regain his equanimity once he was free of administrative duties. He could return to private practice if he desired; but when I mentioned this to him, he seemed indifferent. I found his attitude discouraging because a doctor who doesn't care about his patients doesn't care enough to pick up cues necessary to help them. Still, if Monroe no longer wanted to see patients, he had textbooks in need of revision and articles to write. He could do desk work with or without his leg.

Faithful patients urged Monroe to examine their eyes again. His associates, now incorporated, encouraged him to return to practice. When, eventually, he did, he grumbled because of the difficulties in maneuvering around equipment on his artificial leg.

At my urging, Monroe took up driving again. We bought a larger car with plenty of room. With an automatic transmission he could brake and accelerate with his left foot, so there was no physical problem with his driving.

When he took his driver's test, he went to the Department of Motor Vehicles minus his artificial leg in order to avoid unnecessary explanations. After passing the driver's test, he proceeded to the window where authorization could be obtained for a blue disabled sign. Without looking up from his desk, the clerk asked, "Is your disability temporary or permanent?"

"It's temporary," Monroe responded. "I'm growing a new leg next week."

I jumped for joy. That was my cheerfully sassy Monroe speaking again. It gave me hope for the future.

It was a false hope. I never again heard Monroe's wit come into play. Before long I regretted having urged Monroe to drive.

At the time we took up residence again in Ojai, I bought him a new desk and more bookcases for his library and had loudspeakers installed in it for his music. I was determined to make Monroe happy and on the move again. In looking back, I do not know where I found the energy to do the tasks I set for myself.

Monroe never thanked me for my efforts, which left me hurt and bewildered.

I was told that handicapped people often resent the vitality they see in others. Such information made me worry that I was discouraging Monroe from doing things on his own.

I became increasingly disheartened as summer moved into autumn. At times Monroe showed complete indifference to me; at other times, resentment. I tried hard to understand, to figure out why he rejected me, why he no longer wanted me in bed beside him.

One night I carried a snack to him. The only light in the room came from the television set. As I hastened through the doorway, my foot jammed into the hard base of Monroe's artificial leg which he had dumped onto the shadowed floor. I fell head first against a wall. My head throbbed. My foot pained and puffed and purpled.

Monroe shifted his head to look at the cause of the commotion. Then, without comment, with total indifference, he returned his gaze to the television set. I was too hurt to cry.

Though I limped for the next two weeks, he never asked about my foot. I do not think it was until then that a deep and underlying bitterness began to erode my ability to reason. It made me want to strike out at him. I fought my bitterness daily; I knew how much Monroe had been through. Usually my reason won and I could suppress my resentment; but sometimes a relentless rage consumed me and left me empty with despair.

I tried to analyze Monroe's feelings toward me. I couldn't believe he had forgotten all the dressings I had changed and the medications I had given day after day and night after night. I knew I had pushed him into using crutches instead of letting him sit all day, and I knew I had pushed him from crutches into using an artificial leg and arm canes. I knew he resented my insistence on his being active; but I thought he would thank me—someday when he got better adjusted.

On a trip north we dined with our old friends, Irving and Nora, in a Chinese restaurant. Toward the end of the meal, when the fortune cookies arrived, I broke one open and scanned the pink fortune paper in my hand.

I felt the blood leave my head. I must have paled noticeably, for Nora grabbed the slip from my hand. As she read it, she became frantic, crying out, "There's been a mistake...This wasn't for you... It was meant for somebody else... It's not for you..." But her agitation merely revealed that she, too, had seen the change in Monroe's attitude toward me and that she was doing her best to deny a painful truth.

"He loves you," my fortune declared, "as much as he can, but he cannot love you very much."

Even as it was happening, I couldn't believe that I could be so shaken by a message in a fortune cookie. But I was; and so was Nora; and when Monroe's problem was eventually diagnosed, no scientific description could have said it better.

15

W hile dusting Monroe's desk one day I saw a "Final Notice" on a pile of papers. I couldn't believe it. When we were young we had sometimes received reminders that we were past due, but never a threat from a collection agency.

My parents had taught me that any person's papers are as confidential as medical or legal records. I had never in my life read Monroe's mail unless he passed it on to me.

I could have resisted a perfumed letter, but a final notice was too much. I went through his mail. Along with requests for payments past due were unanswered letters from friends and family and from students asking for recommendations, undeposited checks and unreconciled bank statements. The latter showed we had not only enough money to pay every bill, but an excess that should have been invested.

That night I got Monroe to write checks. In the next two or three days I answered correspondence and authored letters of recommendation for students. I persuaded Monroe to make phone calls regarding urgent letters he had received. I knew he resented my pushing him, but I saw no alternative. In the weeks that followed, I transferred larger and larger amounts from his checking account into my small household account so that I could handle all bills. Monroe never objected to these transfers.

I looked into psychology books and found that not carrying out routine duties is often a sign of depression, but I had no way of confirming my unschooled "diagnosis." Monroe continued to refuse psychiatric care.

When I told people that Monroe seemed depressed, they responded, "Of course he's depressed. I'd be depressed, too, if the same thing happened to me." But a few of us who were close to Monroe were uneasy with this answer.

Following Monroe's routine checkup in late 1978, I told Dr. Tams that Monroe's psychological problem was serious. I asked about the possibility of brain damage. Tarn answered, immediately and emphatically that Methotrexate is not supposed to cross the brain barrier.

I was elated by his answer. My fear of brain damage was banished. I concluded that Monroe might once again become my friend and partner. Sometime later I recalled the incident and remembered that I had not asked him about Methotrexate. I had asked him about brain damage. Why had he talked about Methotrexate? Why had he skimmed past my real questions, my real doubts, my real worries? Was he being defensive?

Perhaps in denying my question, he was denying his doubts. Perhaps in bypassing my question, he was protecting himself. Perhaps in accepting his answer, I was denying my fears. Perhaps I wanted to be talked out of my suspicions. Certainly, I accepted the doctor's reassurance eagerly, and so did my friends. I wanted desperately to be reassured by someone who should know. I never expected to be deceived.

In October, 1978, we attended the dedication of the new optometry wing on the Berkeley campus. After the dedication a sizeable group lunched together. Monroe was seated next to the wife of the chancellor of the university. I was at the next table. Before dessert was served, I heard Monroe's voice rise above the crowd, one obscene or salacious reference following another. The people facing me at his table looked stunned. I got Monroe away from the luncheon as fast as possible.

Monroe had had a cocktail and probably wine during the meal. I thought he must be drunk, but I was puzzled. I had seen him get cheerful on alcohol, but neither vulgar nor incapacitated. I knew he could punctuate a sentence with an expletive, but obscenities never monopolized his talk. I decided that his general abstinence from liquor in the months that followed his cancer surgery had left him unable to handle alcohol. But although that was my conclusion, it worried me. Nothing seemed to add up to a common sense explanation. Nothing fit the man I had known for forty years.

16

Sometime during the summer of 1978 Monroe was invited by the American Academy of Optometry to receive the Prentice Medal, the highest optometric award for contributions to the advancement of knowledge in the visual sciences. He agreed to go to the meeting and give a scientific discourse.

When Monroe told me he would receive the medal, I thought nothing could be better for him than a trip to Boston to receive the honor and be among his scientific colleagues.

He seemed undisturbed about giving a major speech and did nothing to prepare for it. I began to fret to myself that he would extemporize and get lost as he had at his Berkeley farewell party. When he continued to do no work on the speech, I thought of reporting my predicament to the Academy; but I worried what effect my interference would have on his mental state and his feelings toward me. Then, in autumn the printed Academy program arrived with Monroe's speech listed on it. I realized it was too late to cancel. I begged Monroe to work on his lecture.

"I don't know what to talk about," he answered simply. "I haven't done research lately."

I replied that the members knew he had been sick and wouldn't expect recent research. I suggested he retrace the history of the different theories of myopia on which he was an authority. In addition to his own research, he had read over two thousand articles on the subject and summarized their contents on individual cards. I carried the files of these annotated cards to his desk and left them for him.

He worked on the cards for a long time. He laughed and chuckled often. He pulled many cards from his file, but after his first burst of enthusiasm, he left the cards on his desk and didn't return to them. I encouraged him again to work on his speech. Then, as the date of the speech grew close and my anxieties increased, I badgered him. Nothing worked.

A week before we were to leave for the December meeting, I thought again of canceling the speech but feared my doing so would deepen Monroe's resentment against me. I was well aware that the Academy was not a place to speak without careful preparation. The knots in my stomach tightened and I tripled my antacid intake.

Panic gripped me the next time I noticed the cards in their untouched piles. I began to sob, but Monroe remained indifferent.

With no one to encourage my self-pity, I wiped my eyes and blew my nose and tried to collect myself. I began to inspect the cards Monroe had put into two separate piles. The smaller pile contained sound evidence that non-pathological eye defects are almost always hereditary. The other pile contained bizarre, often contradictory theories, the "evidence" for which was utterly irrational to anyone with minimal scientific knowledge. These cards were so ridiculous that I began to laugh. Then I realized that these were the cards that had made Monroe laugh as he pulled them.

Soon I was playing with the cards. I began to arrange them so that absurd "evidence" used to support one theory lay in opposition to contrary and equally absurd statements used to support another theory. One of these impossible theories held that gravity caused the eyeball to elongate and, hence, become nearsighted if children were permitted to lie on their stomachs while reading the funny papers. I was personally familiar with that theory because my parents insisted that I sit erect while doing close work so that I would not become nearsighted. Because of that theory, I always sat up while reading, but I became nearsighted anyway.

I had worked so many years with Monroe and absorbed so much of his thinking that as I played with the cards I began to formulate the speech indicated by the pulled cards. I began to think how he would say his speech and how funny he would make it, and before long, I began to type it. As I typed, I realized it was more like an after-dinner speech than a scientific contribution; but I could only risk being an editor, not an original scientist. When it was honed and completed a couple of days later, I gave it to Monroe. He said it was a very good speech.

On the day of the speech itself, my stomach felt like a hot stone. I did not know whether Monroe would use the speech I had written. If he did use it, I did not know whether that would be good or bad. If he read the speech I had ghosted, would it pass inspection by the professors and the brainiest practitioners in the audience? I could barely believe that a man such as Monroe would accept a ghostwritten speech and read it as his own. But that is exactly what he did. He did not deviate from the speech by one iota.

Everyone applauded his speech, more because of Monroe, I'm sure, than for the speech itself. It was not as strong, as original, or as authoritative as Monroe would once have made it, but it was accurate and polished, and it was amusing. It was even, I heard one doctor say, "splendid."

One person after another came up to Monroe with happy grins on their faces to say how glad they were that his sickness had not curbed his sense of humor.

My deception had passed the test.

One more crisis was behind us.

17

My father had loved all the trappings of Christmas from the yule log to the Christmas tree to the stuffed turkey which he himself carved at the head of the table. There was no opening of presents the night before Christmas or early in the morning. As a courtesy to my mother, he insisted we appear at the breakfast table on time, completely dressed and groomed. In this respect, Christmas was no different than any other day. But on Christmas morning, instead of bacon and eggs, we had oatmeal, and until everyone finished his oatmeal, there were no festivities.

Some people might see a touch of sadism in this arrangement. Whether there was or not, it was terrific showmanship. By the time the red velvet draperies were drawn back slowly between the living room and the music room to expose the tree in all its decorated glory, everyone under ten had peed in his pants in an ecstasy of excitement.

After my father died, I was the member of our family who most identified with his childlike and sentimental love of Christmas tradition. It was to our house that some of Monroe's family and all of mine usually came to celebrate.

I was determined that the holidays of 1978 would be happy, especially for Monroe. But on December 23, the day before the family was expected, I was swept into a rage beyond restraint of reason. By the time my wrath was exhausted, I despised myself. I believed I had wounded Monroe so deeply he would retreat farther and farther within himself.

I had brought home two tricycles for our grandsons. I bought them unassembled because Monroe had liked to work with his hands; assembling tricycles would give him the same kind of satisfaction he got from solving a puzzle. I was proud of myself for creating a situation that would make Monroe happy.

I laid out the tricycle parts and the necessary tools and supplies. He became as engrossed in working on the tricycles as he had in pulling cards for his Prentice Award speech.

Meanwhile, I prepared for houseguests, hid toys and extended the table so that everyone could sit together for dinner. The next day I would have the turkey to stuff and the guests to receive and all the chores a housewife runs into before a feast day.

As the day ended, I was worn out. I looked at the tricycles Monroe had put together and began to compliment him. Then I stopped, for although the tricycles looked complete at first glance, there were parts left over. Monroe had worked from memory of tricycle mechanics, but he had not followed the instruction which came with the toys. He had not followed such cautions as "be sure to get the seat in place before the pedals."

Each pedal was held firmly in place by a cap with teeth hammered onto the pedal bar. Once hammered in place, the teeth bent in such a way as to prevent the cap from falling off.

With the cap hammered into the bar, there was no easy way to fit the seat rod to the pedal bar.

At first I was merely annoyed that Monroe hadn't followed instructions. Then, when he refused to correct the errors I grew angry; and when I tried to pry apart the tricycles in order to repair them and realized it would be a major effort and that I still had a hundred things to do of my own, my anger went out of control. I carried on to Monroe about all the things I had to do without having to undo a couple of tricycles. And I told him that if he weren't so damn conceited he would have known he had to follow instructions, and I couldn't imagine how he could ever do anything so damn dumb.

He answered simply, "I did it so dumb because I'm dumb. You think I'm dumb."

Shocked by his answer, but not shocked enough to reduce my wrath or to lower my voice to a reasonable level, I raged that I didn't think he was dumb, that I had never said he was dumb, but it was still a damn dumb thing to do. I grumbled the evening away, pulling apart the tricycles and putting them together again.

If I had used my brains instead of my adrenals, I would have thrown the tricycles out and replaced them after Christmas.

If I had known in 1978 what someone would explain to me in 1980, I would not have ranted at Monroe. I would never have given him a task his brain could no longer handle. I would have loved Monroe as I found him instead of struggling to regain for him what could no longer be.

18

M ike, Monroe's partner, was as bewildered by Monroe's performance in the optometric office as I was by his behavior with me. Some patients were satisfied; others were not. They took their complaints to Mike. He decided to go over Monroe's clinical records to find out what was going wrong.

Mike found that Monroe never made an error in the tests he did. He was still an outstandingly competent refractionist; but once he had finished an examination, he no longer succeeded with complex prescriptions or bothered to finish tests that were physically difficult for him to do. He did not explain his results to his patients as he had formerly done, and he was abrupt with them.

With malpractice uppermost in their minds, his partners urged him to work more carefully and patiently, but he brushed them aside. They did not bother me about their worries for quite some time. Instead, they followed after him, making sure that his patients received proper care. Ultimately, they became baffled by Monroe's curtness and contrariness when they were doing their utmost to encourage him, and a rage against Monroe began to build within them. Sometimes I saw the same fury on their faces as that which burned inside me. But in 1978 they understood no better than I why Monroe acted unreasonably because no professional person had admitted that something more than depression was involved.

I found out later that the cause of Monroe's irresponsible actions was severe damage to the frontal lobes of his brain. A psychometric evaluation on Monroe dated October 24, 1980, explains that "The 'frontal lobe' patient... cannot and does not use his intellect to solve his problems... Although frontal lobe patients are frequently seen by others as being depressed, true depression is seldom found... the patient looks depressed over losses revolving around job, family and personal relationships, etc., but is not truly depressed..."

Such patients exhibit "profound personality change, lack of tact, foresight, insight or concern, inability to judge consequences of one's own actions and behavior..."

"Qualitatively, the patient makes mistakes characteristic of frontal lobe impairment: impulsive, concrete, stereotyped responses. They make no attempt to correct obvious mistakes..." His intellect, however, was "relatively intact."

As I read the evaluation, each phrase brought to mind an action of Monroe's that had disturbed and baffled me and for which I had no explanation at the time. It helped me understand how he could write checks and enter them into his account book but failed to reconcile his bank statement. It helped me understand how he could select interesting information for a lecture but failed to synthesize it. It helped me understand how he was able to put together a tricycle from memory but could not correct his errors. It helped me understand how he could prescribe lenses for a patient whose problem was simple but failed to successfully prescribe if an eye problem was complicated.

Even as I read that Monroe's intelligence was still above average though "below what should be expected from past achievements," my mind flashed to a time before we were married. I had phoned him and was surprised to find him abrupt. He announced he would see me in an hour; then the receiver clicked off.

When he came over an hour later, he was chuckling and puffed up with amused pride. One of his roommates, a psychology major with a lot of insecurity problems, was learning to give intelligence tests. He had asked Monroe to be a subject for his practice testing. Monroe was to answer as many questions as possible within a limited time.

My telephone call came while Monroe was being tested. Over the protests of the psychology major, Monroe answered the phone and returned to complete the test within the allotted time. When the test was corrected, the psychology major was furious. Nobody, according to the instruction sheet, could do as well as Monroe had done. Monroe was elated, not only with the results of the test, but because he didn't care very much for the psychology major.

It is not fair either to Monroe or to me that I continue his story without re-affirming that he had lost the power of volitional control and that I did not know what had happened to Monroe's brain until late in 1980. If I had known it, I could have protected both of us from sharp misunderstandings and painful situations. If I had also known that with frontal lobe dysfunction comes a "coarsening of personality," I could have avoided the fiercest grief of all—the grief that comes from alienation and rejection by the one I loved.

I first noticed this "coarsening," this grossness, in Monroe after we sold our Berkeley house in 1978. We had moved into a furnished house until Monroe's contract with the university ended. In the bookshelves Monroe found a few books on marriage with emphasis on methods of physical coupling. Sexual enlightenment, I recognized, can be obtained from texts, but Monroe displayed a morbid fascination with these books. He often roamed the house at night because phantom pains in the stump of his leg kept him awake. If I wakened, I found him poring over these books, strangely absorbed.

I had read that loss of a leg tends to be more traumatic for men than for women because they often associate it with castration and feel less than men because of it. I thought Monroe's abnormal concentration on these books was a fear of failure during intercourse. I tried to show Monroe my love and confidence in him. If he bothered to respond at all, it was with rejection.

I began to feel hopeful when I heard noises of a person enjoying sexual pleasure from Monroe's room. It may seem strange that a wife would rejoice at sounds of masturbation, but I thought Monroe had found he was a man again and would soon realize he was as competent to give sexual pleasure as he had been before. I found comfort in the old maxim that a person doesn't think sex if he does sex.

Sometime during the summer of 1979 I hired Bill, a thirteen-year-boy to work for me. Bill washed the car willingly, cleaned the yard, and helped himself to the ice cream in our refrigerator.

One day Bill brought a friend to help. Monroe was on his bed in the little room, and the friend had gone into the bathroom in the hall adjacent to it. By mistake he had locked himself into the bathroom and could not get out. He called for help. Bill and I, doubled up with mirth at his predicament, came to his rescue. I knew the master key hung in a closet in the same hallway as the bathroom and the little room. But before I could reach it, I heard Monroe moaning for a sweetheart, a lover, a baby doll. Instead of getting the key, I crashed against the door of the little room, pretending I had tripped and fallen.

I do not know if my action diverted the boys' attention, but from then on I knew I must never let anyone be within earshot of Monroe unless I could intervene before his fantasies grew audible.

I reported the incident to a psychologist I had begun to see. He evidenced no concern about it.

19

Feelings between Monroe and me had become so strained by 1979 that I felt I would explode unless I could defuse my rages and stop the pain of bereavement over the love I had lost. As the barrier between Monroe and me seemed more and more impregnable with each passing day, my frustrated need for him reached self-murdering proportions

I asked Monroe to get psychiatric care. I begged him to get it, and I raged at him because he would not.

Though almost consumed by my frustrations, I nevertheless realized they were destroying not only me but the Monroe-who-once-loved me. It was then I began to write out my rage. I began to write out my feelings and my grievances and let my pain flow into ink and from ink into oblivion.

A few of my jottings escaped the trash barrel. Their only worth is that I divulged to the privacy of my pen the things that were too painful to confide to people made of flesh and blood.

On January 27, 1979, one year from the day when Monroe's leg broke, I wrote:

"It has been a terrible year... The shock of losing his leg has been too great for him. He's so far from the irrepressibly eager young man who entered my heart so many years ago that I weep and wonder, worry and weep. I know it does no good, but I can hold myself together no longer, at least not always, not every day, not all day long."

On January 29 my scribblings were agitated and hard to read: "Rage at his indolence does no good. I feel sick all over from holding my rage against him. But what can I do? Rage at him succeeds not a bit in moving him out of self-pity, self-torture, or whatever it is that is destroying him. Is he worried that he still has cancer? Does every tiny ache or pain alarm him about a return of cancer? I do not know. I do believe that if I entertained the idea that cancer was about to destroy me, I would want to live each second to the hilt. But if it really happened to me would I so respond? Or would I feed and feed and feed upon my worries and weaknesses and so destroy myself by slow torture? I don't know..."

On the morning of January 30 I pulled a box from the top shelf of a closet, put there before we migrated to Berkeley. That day I wrote: "It doesn't seem much to write about—a pair of shoes. But I felt so tender toward Monroe when I found them in the box. The bows were still tied, laced so tightly that the tongue did not show between the sides. He had always done that—just wriggled into and out of his shoes without every untying them. He had such a slender foot."

February 2: "Robin came yesterday when I was feeling blue. I almost told her that I planned to move away from Monroe, that I thought my absence might make him achieve again. But I didn't. I can't quite face it yet, although I must..."

February 5: "I broached the subject (to Monroe) of moving to another place—not because I didn't love him, but because we were no longer good for each other. I said that if he preferred, he could be the one to move. He responded: 'I will move out on you. I will go up and live with Jeff. They still have an empty room!'

How dependent he has become! So unlike his former self."

In every way I was treating Monroe as a person with a functioning brain, as one who could love his friends and family but was feeling too sorry for himself to care about us. I was treating him as one who could cope with the problems of a household and of the world but whose illness had depressed him to the point of not functioning as he had before.

Try as I would to be kind to Monroe and succeed as a I did much of the time, my resentment against his self-centered acts sometimes burst into shrieks of rage or streams of tears.

On my birthday I took Monroe with me to the store to buy binoculars for bird watching. He could make a better selection than I because of his knowledge of optics. Besides, I hoped for a present from him.

I parked in front of the store, but Monroe refused to accompany me inside. I entered alone, but he followed immediately. Then, instead of going to the binocular counter, he went to the window at the front of the store. I carried a pair of binoculars to him and asked if they were good. He didn't answer, but turned to glare at me with undisguised hatred. Blinded by tears, I paid as fast as I could for the binoculars in my hand, the only ones I had had a chance to look at.

To cry at home was bad enough, but to display my hurt in public was more than I could bear.

I think often of birthdays past and of Monroe bearing gifts to me, even when there was no special occasion. And I have laughed at a birthday forgotten. A long time ago Monroe received a letter from a relative who complained that Monroe had not remembered her birthday. Monroe made immediate amends. He selected greeting cards for Halloween, Thanksgiving, Chanukah, Christmas, Valentine's, Passover, Easter, birthday and St. Patrick's Day. He bundled them off to her with the hope that she would not feel neglected for the rest of the year.

On March 2, 1979, Monroe had a routine checkup at the oncologists' office. I was in the waiting room when Dr. Tarns walked up to say that a lump had appeared on Monroe's stump and Monroe must have a biopsy. I wept suddenly and desperately, this time for myself as well as for Monroe. I knew not how I could take care of Monroe during another recovery with no thanks, no love, no appreciation.

And I wept, too, becuase Tarns allowed my distress to be exhibited in public. Surely he could have told me the distressing news in the privacy of his office.

The lump proved to be non-cancerous. We were told to come back in July.

20

In May, 1979, I took Monroe to the Los Angeles airport. He was on his way to Chicago to receive an Honorary Doctor of Science from the Illinois College of Optometry. I had rationalized that it would be better for Monroe to go without me, that it would help if he were free of the tensions between us. But in reality I was terrified of going to another meeting with him. I could no longer deny that sooner or later I would have to see my idol fall and that when he did, I could not stand to watch it. So, I let him go alone.

Before long word trickled back to me that Monroe had been insulting to his sponsors and had barely managed a "thank you." Those who had come to honor Monroe were indignant.

The person who told me loved Monroe and wanted me to apologize for Monroe's rudeness and for my not being present to keep things running smoothly. I was dreadfully upset, but I did nothing. I didn't know what to do. I didn't know what to say. No explanation for Monroe's behavior had ever been given to me.

By spring, 1979, I was crying too easily, too frequently, but not for long at a time.

In the summer I woke one day before dawn and began to cry, and my tears would not stop. I could no longer promise myself that by forbidding myself to weep I could control myself enough to get through the day.

I told Monroe truthfully that I needed professional help; then I enticed him into coming with me to a psychologist's office to show how we responded to each other.

Monroe glowered as I recited my worries to the psychologist who shall go by the name of Button. I begged Monroe to join the discussion and quarrelled with him because he would not. The more Monroe remained silent and hostile, the more I talked. I couldn't stop talking and complaining and beseeching. It was a horrible confrontation. I did not want to behave that way, but I did. My feelings had burst my control.

Monroe had often praised me for suppressing whatever quarrel I might be engaged in if a third party appeared. He said I had never embarrassed him with recriminations. But there, in the presence of the psychologist, I found fault without let-up. It was obvious that I needed help, too.

I made an appointment to see Dr. Button again. Monroe refused. He said Button was too young to know anything. That was so unlike my old Monroe, the one who had appreciated and encouraged young people.

The first time I saw Button alone I told him how important it was to help Monroe. Button reminded me that Monroe was not present to be helped; that I was there to be helped, which, in turn, might help Monroe.

I had several sessions with Button. Whenever he directed the discussion to me, I must have talked about Monroe. Button soon complained that I never spoke of "me"— that I spoke only of "us." He said he had never seen two lives so intertwined, that he could not keep the threads apart.

Guessing that he admired Kahlil Gibran, I quoted: "But let there be spaces in your togetherness, and let the winds of the heavens dance between you."

He perked up and asked, "How do you feel about that?"

I responded that only the success of a marriage could hint at the proper ingredients. To myself I wondered how many people who began marriage with spaces between each other would achieve thirty-eight years of meaningful happiness as Monroe and I had before our lives began to fall apart.

It was true that our thirty-ninth year had been agonizing, but I knew that if we were to begin our lives together again, I would not change the symbiotic relationship we had developed, even if I could.

One time I told Button that I tried not to let Monroe see me cry because he didn't like it.

Button asked me where I went to cry.

"In my room or on the woodpile behind the garage." And I almost added, "Out in the cemetery," but checked myself. If I had told him that, he would have asked, with carefully concealed concern, that I might be suicidal, "Why the cemetery?"

My honest answer would have been, "Because I needed someone to talk to." If I had said that, he would have thought me crazy.

I told Button of Monroe's recent failure to invest our money wisely. I told him I had let Monroe keep these tasks because he had been proud of his ability to handle financial matters and I did not want to do anything that would push Monroe farther down. I probably didn't admit to Button how incompetent I was at handling money.

Monroe had always known to the penny how much money we had. I neither understood bookkeeping nor considered it relevant as long as I had money in my purse. Consequently, I was rarely entrusted with the books when I worked in Monroe's office. One December, however, we were short of help and Monroe was attending a convention, so I kept the accounts. Payments coming into the office exceeded our needs, so I not only paid every bill on the day it arrived, I was overly generous with Christmas gifts.

Upon his return I greeted him with the news that we were well ahead financially. He looked surprised, said nothing, but inspected the books as soon as we got to work the next morning. "You've made a thousand dollar error!" he blazed. "How could you make a mistake like that?"

"It was easy," I answered, perhaps too cheerfully. "I added wrong..."

"You added wrong! You've overdrawn the checking account! You should have sensed..."

Monroe's failure to appreciate my efforts threw me into a passion and I screamed, "You're not fair! You're using logic—and that's really not fair in a fight!"

Monroe choked with laughter at my accusation. Then, to humor my hurt feelings, he said, "It's OK. Everyone knows it's as easy to add wrong in the thousand column as it is in the penny column. "But," I heard him mumble to himself, "they'll never believe it at the bank when I try to tell them what happened."

Dr. Button let me know that I had been too dependent on my husband and that I must assume responsibility in our financial affairs. He was still too young, too unaware of the world, I'm sure, to realize that his advice would involve me in corporation papers, partnership agreements, a marital agreement, wills, income tax, fine print in insurance policies, rollover pension plans and a buy-sell agreement. I was so ignorant of the marketplace and so oriented toward science that, when my attorney told me to locate a "buy-sell" agreement for him, I hunted for papers headed "bi-cell."

Button advanced the idea that my close attachment to Monroe had acted like tendrils suffocating him. I should give Monroe "space."

Button thought the amputation was associated with castration in Monroe's mind. He shuddered his own reaction when he said, "After all, it was close."

He apparently assigned little importance to my statements about Monroe's fantasizing. If he had, he might have looked deeper into Monroe's problem than a lost leg and a suffocating wife. Button gave me the impression that he thought me sexually repressed, skittish about masculine needs, the frigid stereotype of females of my vintage. I told him he was wrong, but he didn't appear to accept that. I stopped protesting. It was enough for me that I knew I had never denied myself to Monroe, not out of any sense of duty, but because I loved to have his body couched with mine. At no time did Button reflect the possibility that Monroe's's fantasizing might be neurological and entirely beyond his or my influence.

Friends have criticized Button for not suggesting a brain scan for Monroe. He should have, but few people have insight beyond their own specialities and beyond the clues fed them. Had Button known of an episode that took place shortly after Monroe's amputation, he might have called for a brain scan.

Not until a year later did someone ask the question that uncovered a clue which had been withheld from me. It was a clue, I believe, I was never expected to find.

By the time I said farewell to Button on my last visit and in spite of a non-solution of Monroe's problem, my own emotional strength was greatly improved. I had been helped by unburdening my sorrows on someone. I came away determined to give Monroe more space and to develop interests of my own. The more interests I developed, the more interesting I would become to others. And the more interesting I became, the more I could bring exciting stories home to Monroe. I would be able to reciprocate with entertaining tidbits for the lively stories Monroe had once brought home from work to me.

Or so I thought.

21

In the summer of 1979 I obtained a portable wheelchair for Monroe. During a routine trip to the oncology group, Dr. Tarns asked why Monroe needed a wheelchair. I explained that we could go through museums and art exhibits and other big buildings more easily, that if Monroe got out more often, his mental state might improve.

On the next routine visit I caught Tarns in the waiting room and asked if he would write a prescription for a pill to make Monroe more cheerful. I told Tarns that if Monroe could become more cheerful, maybe he could be talked into seeing a psychologist. Tarns prescribed Elavil. It didn't seem to help Monroe.

In looking back, I'm sure I never left any doubt in Tarn's mind that Monroe's mental condition was not only paramount to me but that I was doing my utmost to understand it and to cope with it.

No matter how hard I tried to treat it lightly, Monroe's fantasizing besieged me with apprehension and feelings of inadequacy. I had never known jealously before; but with his phantom lover, Monroe was oblivious of me, and I could neither outwit her nor kill her nor tolerate her. I could only run from her.

I had Monroe's big bed moved to his library where he could sleep and read and watch television without me. But even with the door shut I could hear him in the next room calling to his imaginary lover, and I could not stand it. I retreated to the little room at the other end of the house and turned it into my sitting room and study. I stopped encouraging friends to drop by. I stopped answering the door chimes unless I was sure no sounds of endearment were coming from the library. If I let a visitor in, I did not let him dally. I gave Monroe the freedom of the house. I took him on excursions every day, but I barred the outside world from entering our doors as much as I was able.

On an office visit early in 1980 I again caught Tarns in the waiting room and told him that Monroe was in desperate need of mental help and that he would listen to no doctor but Tarns. I begged him to obtain psychiatric care for Monroe.

After Tarns examined Monroe and found no evidence of cancer spread, he sped past me in the waiting room and announced that he told Monroe to see a psychiatrist.

Monroe needed more than an admonition. Monroe needed to be institutionalized so that he could be studied; but for that I needed help, real help. I needed someone to force the issue with Monroe. Tarns, it appeared was not the one who would do it. Leadened with despair, I drove Monroe home to Ojai.

22

As we had in years past, we celebrated the arrival of 1980 with our old friends, Irving and Nora, at a beach resort.

Monroe stayed in his room as Irving and Nora and I walked to the stairway leading down to Shell Beach. Irving wasted no time in asking about Monroe's hostility to me. I confessed that Monroe hadn't said a kind word to me in months, that he rarely spoke to me at all. I told him about my birthday when Monroe had refused to help me select binoculars.

Nora continued on her way. She seemed to sense that Irving and I needed to be by ourselves in our bewilderment and despair.

I can see Irving still, his arm resting on a railing high above the sea, the wind raising the remnants of his once red hair. Tears welled in his eyes. "But I don't understand... You took good care of him. Doesn't he remember?"

I shrugged off the good care. I had become a chamber-maid, nothing more. Kisses don't come with the job.

Four months later Nora phoned to say that Irving had died with no sign of struggle against the heart attack that killed him. "He loved and cared for you," she added, perhaps to fill the numb void at my end of the line. "I know," I managed to respond. "I loved him, too."

My confidant, my staunchest ally was dead. I no longer had a shoulder I could cry on.

I left Monroe in Ojai to attend Irving's memorial service. It was exactly forty years earlier that Monroe and I, eloping to Vallejo, discovered that Irving had stowed away in the rumble seat of the car. He waited until we passed the toll gate of the Carquinez Bridge before he lifted the rumble seat cover under which he had hidden. Then he thumbed his nose merrily at the toll collector for having missed a fare. He announced that we couldn't elope without him.

Was it possible that we were ever so young?

The next day I visited Jeff and Francia. It is difficult to convince young people that death in the manner of Irving is better than life in the manner of Monroe. Young people are not the only ones who fail to understand this. Physicians fail, too. I think physicians on the whole are more comfortable prolonging a deadly life than giving ground to a kindly death.

By the time I saw Jeff and Francia, I was in control of the family finances. It had taken me a long time to assume this responsibility, not only because I was terrified of accounting, but because I didn't know how to acquire our joint investments.

Because no doctor had admitted incapacity on Monroe's part, Monroe would have to give consent in order for me to become his conservator. Our attorney had been Monroe's patient since high school. Both of us knew how Monroe prided himself on his skill with numbers. Both of us came close to tears at the idea of taking financial control from Monroe through a conservatorship. Both of us feared Monroe's mental health would deteriorate as a result.

Finally, although I was told it would not hold in court, we decided to try a marital agreement. It would be painless if Monroe agreed. It consisted simply of dividing our investments into three parts: His, Hers, and Ours, to be managed as the names implied. Even if Monroe neglected his portion, we would be better off than if no one was improving some of our investments.

Monroe did not object as we divided our properties. The divisions were very much along the lines he had made before he was sick, and he said it was time to put our finances in order.

As I worked on the division of our properties, my appreciation for Monroe increased. Though I had paid little attention to his investments, I now found he had shared with me always. Only items relating to the optometric practice were in his name. Only stocks given me by my parents were in mine.

I found he had been so considerate of me that he had put in writing his exact wishes for the disposal of his body after death. The only thing he had neglected to do was write down his beliefs against extending his life if death would be less cruel.

23

Vaguely, almost from the time we married, I had sensed that some day I might pay dearly for establishing few interests beyond Monroe and his activities. So it was not surprising that as Monroe dropped out of optometry which I loved and as he dropped out of the academic world which I loved and as he withdrew into his own world which I could not enter, I found myself cut off from the people and discussions I had most enjoyed.

The simple expedient of phoning old friends to unburden myself was out of the question. As long as I believed that any comments about Monroe's physical or mental health would deepen his "depression," I could not speak within his hearing. I came to dread calls from relatives asking what was being done to help Monroe, what the doctor was doing to end his depression, when would Monroe have his next cancer check. I did not know how to answer them so that Monroe would not worry about my answers. Sometimes I went to homes of friends to make phone calls to doctors and relatives, but that was awkward, too.

I could no longer welcome people to our home, so I made no effort to acquire new friends. I knew I should keep contact with the outside world, so I tried to find new niches, ones without social obligations.

I volunteered to do clerical work in the office of the local senior citizens organization. Aside from answering five or six phone calls during an afternoon, there was little to keep me busy in that job. It gave me no sense of worth. Instead, it increased my loneliness and made me feel too old to do anything but busywork.

I dropped out of that job but studied how to help elderly people fill income tax forms. I never felt comfortable taking responsibility for other people's tax forms, but I improved the management of our own finances.

I learned that the local museum needed senior volunteers. With postgraduate studies in anthropology in my background, I thought my knowledge might be useful. When I applied, the man in charge of the museum welcomed me to sit at the entrance way and answer the phone. To my reply that I was seeking more active tasks, he responded tactlessly, "So bring your knitting. That's what the other old ladies do."

Finding more comfort in nature than in the groups I had approached, I began taking longer and longer walks. I indulged myself in a fisherman's vest. With its six zippered pockets and pouch on back, I could walk with binoculars, keys and driver's license and let my arms swing free.

One pocket was reserved for handkerchiefs because I was often overcome by sudden tears. Sometimes the tears were for a moment of intense beauty that I could no longer share with Monroe. Sometimes the tears were from fear that Monroe was beyond hope. I had read that the longer a person remains depressed, the less likely it is that mental health will be restored. By 1980, most of our friends assumed that Monroe was depressed. His "depression" had lasted two years.

I woke one morning in the spring of 1980, luxuriated in the warmth of my own body, turned over and went back to sleep. I had not wakened and begun to cry. One phase of bitter "widowhood" was over. I had learned to wake up alone.

24

On May 3, 1980, during a routine visit to the oncology group, I was seated in the waiting room when Dr. Tarns approached with two young men in tow. They both wore white laboratory coats and kept a respectful distance behind him. They were probably interns being educated by the master. Tarns assured me with widening grin that my husband's mental health was fine. "You've no worry. Monroe just gave me...," he paused and chuckled in the direction of his acolytes, "he just gave me a vulgar gesture! Monroe's just fine." And with that he was off, his wing-tipped shoes leading the way, the two young men still at a discreet distance behind him.

I was stunned. That Tarns could consider an upthrust middle finger as a definitive sign of normal behavior was stupid, especially for Monroe, who had been quite capable of meaningful epithets if the occasion called for it. That Tarns would pass off Monroe's gesture as a diagnosis of sound mental condition to two "interns" was horrendous, even if done in jest, and that he would consider me so prudish that he had to titter about "a vulgar gesture" was condescending. I found myself wishing the doctor's brains were in his feet which were outsized and always in the lead.

I found myself wondering, not for the first time, why Monroe was content to keep Tarns as his physician. He was completely unlike the colleagues or students Monroe had most respected and admired, the ones who thought before they spoke, the ones whose thinking added up.

Unfortunately, in that spring of 1980 I had not yet been told that Monroe's ability to judge was gone. In deference to Monroe's training and the judgment I thought Monroe still had, I made small effort to argue him into seeking health care elsewhere.

Then, too, I didn't know where else to go. Would another oncology group take him? If so, would that group be any better? Would the change depress Monroe? Would Monroe resent me more? The problem seemed too overwhelming at the time, so I let things drift.

At about this same time, Monroe was the driver in three automobile accidents in as many months. He had not told me about the last accident when a man came to our door demanding the name of our insurance agent.

I supplied him with the information. The man said Monroe had braked at a stop sign as his own car began to pass in front of Monroe. Suddenly, Monroe's car leaped forward and struck his. The man suggested that the device we had on the car to enable Monroe to drive with only one leg had apparently snapped and caused the car to go out of control. The man left, content with the knowledge that our insurance would take care of his car and his own injury, which was slight.

I was shocked that Monroe had told me nothing about the accident and the man's being hurt. I was distressed that Monroe didn't seem to care that he had caused pain and inconvenience. He didn't seem to appreciate how kind the man had been to offer the excuse of a special driving mechanism—a mechanism which the car didn't have. None had been necessary because, with an automatic transmission, all Monroe had to do was use his left foot instead of his missing right foot to brake or accelerate.

I was in the car at the time of Monroe's first accident, and the sequence of events was the same: a stop at an intersection and an acceleration into the street too abrupt to allow the slow-travelling car in front of us to pass by.

After the last accident I asked Monroe for the keys to his car. He protested. I promised him that I would return the keys if he would see a psychiatrist and the psychiatrist approved of his driving. Monroe refused to see a psychiatrist and he stopped driving.

Taking the keys to a man's car is no way to gain his affection.

Listing Monroe's erratic driving as a symptom of mental disturbance does not receive serious consideration from anybody. Don't all old ladies carp about their husband's driving?

25

By early summer, 1980, life in my small portion of Ojai had become unadulterated hell.

My brother was put in my care while his wife was hospitalized. He had had a stroke from which he had only partially recovered. The day I met my brother at the airport was the first day of the hottest and longest heat wave in my memory. My brother couldn't stand to be left alone or have others left alone. He became distraught if we went out in the car and left Monroe behind, even if Monroe wanted to stay home.

My mother had a series of small strokes and had to be moved to a convalescent hospital.

I had so many tasks I was in motion from early morning until midnight. I had gone without help inside the house because of Monroe's fantasizing, but a middle-aged woman whom I liked very much offered to clean for us. She was intelligent, an immigrant. She worked as a maid in a house at the edge of the Los Padres Forest. She had seen me weeping on the forest road when she drove to work in the morning. She was grateful to Monroe because he had helped get her son into medical school. She knew I was overworked and over worried. She admired Monroe. She offered to help me and insisted she could spare an hour or two a week to help us out.

I knew from past experience that Isabella, as I shall call her, could do better work in an hour than most people do in a day. She was vivacious and cheerful and would help out in the middle of the afternoon at a time when Monroe was usually quiescent. She was so insistent and I was so desperate for help that I agreed.

On the day she came to work, she arrived late; but she rolled up her sleeves and elected to clean the library where Monroe lay on his bed watching television. I heard her talking to him as I was called to the phone. Then I started dinner.

After an hour Isabella left with a hurried good-bye. The library glistened from her brief attack upon it. The next time she was due for work, she didn't arrive. I was disappointed and thought of telephoning but decided not to bother her. I felt sure she had a good reason for missing her time with us, and I was correct.

She telephoned two days later, nervous and upset. In broken English her words leaped together telling me she knew I would be angry with her but after being so very upset thinking about it she had told her son what had happened and he said she must tell Mrs. Hirsch because Dr. Hirsch was a very sick man. Isabella began to cry and said she knew I didn't know how Monroe acted and she tried not to notice, but was so embarrassed and please not to hate her even if I didn't understand and she didn't know how to tell me what he did, but she didn't want to work for us any more.

I thanked Isabella, sickened though I was at what she told me. I assured her that I knew what Monroe had done and she needn't tell me more. I said I was aware that Monroe was a very sick man but I hadn't found a doctor who would agree with me. I promised I would use the information she had given me to get help for Monroe's mind.

I hung up the receiver perhaps more hastily than I should have, but I was sick with shame and worry. Not knowing where else to turn, I phoned an old friend, a reporter for a local newspaper. She had come to our house to interview Monroe about the Prentice Medal he had won. A few days later she commented to me on how much his personality had changed since he lost his leg. She mentioned that she had a good friend, a woman psychologist with a Ph.D. who might help.

After the phone call from Isabella I sought and obtained her assistance immediately.

26

As a favor to us, the psychologist met us at night after she was home from her regular job. The date was August 10, 1980.

During her conference with me, Dr. Lorraine (not her real name) stated the seriousness of Monroe's lack of control in front of Isabella. She indicated that loss of a limb could cause deep depression; but, she said, the symptoms indicated a neurological origin. She added, after more questions and answers, that everything I said pointed to the amputation as the time the change in Monroe took place. Suddenly she asked if anything had happened at the time of the amputation that seemed to be wrong. Did anything strange happen during the surgery?

Just as suddenly my mind played back an entire scene which had occurred, not during surgery, but shortly thereafter. I was standing next to the elevator in the private ward of the hospital when the door opened. Monroe was wheeled out on a gurney. He was accompanied by a man in operating room regalia.

I expressed surprise when Monroe was taken into the room reserved for him rather than into the intensive care section which lay directly opposite. The gentleman accompanying Monroe introduced himself. He told me that he was the anesthesiologist and that my husband had gone through surgery well.

After he left I stayed in the room with Monroe; but the light was bad because it was late in the afternoon. Monroe was slumbering and I did not wish to disturb him. I wished to work on my needlepoint, so I moved thirty paces away from Monroe's room to a small alcove where the light was better.

Some time later, bells rang and feet scurried past me in the hall. I heard the strong voice of a man yell, "God damn it! I told you not to do that!"

Suddenly a man in a white coat rushed in, touched me and asked if my husband snored. As I responded that he did, he turned and shot out the door. I remained in my seat, frozen. I realized it was Monroe who was in trouble. I began to get up. As I did so, the man returned and assured me that Monroe would be all right. He disappeared before I could ask what had happened. When I looked at Monroe, he seemed to be sleeping comfortably. Everything seemed all right and the alarm dropped out of my thoughts. I was only reminded of it again by Lorraine's question.

"Did the man mention Cheyne-Stokes respiration?" She wanted to know. The man had mentioned snoring; but as soon as Lorraine said "Cheyne-Stokes," my mind registered "death rattle." It had never occurred to me that the "rattle" could sound like snoring. It can, and does.

My sudden recall startled me into a new awareness: Something could have happened to Monroe in that hospital room which changed the way he would behave. Deep depression might not be the answer at all.

The next day Dr. Lorraine forced Monroe to act. She insisted in a strongly worded letter that Monroe have a neurological consultation in order "to rule out or accommodate organic influence." The letter needled Monroe into making an appointment with a psychiatrist in Ventura, a nearby city. I shall name him Dr. Campbell.

Two weeks later, Monroe and I were in Dr. Campbell's office. He read Lorraine's letter and wasted no time in saying that Monroe's behavior in front of Isabella was a serious symptom and that we should make a determined effort to seek its cause. I said that was why we were there and that was why Lorraine had suggested a brain scan. With that, he set up an appointment to see Monroe again; but it was useless. Monroe refused to cooperate with Campbell.

For that reason I met with Dr. Campbell on September 9. We discussed Monroe's symptoms again and we both agreed that Monroe must have a brain scan. I mentioned to Campbell that Monroe had a routine oncology appointment with Dr. Tarns in three days. I explained that Monroe had believed that the history of a patient was such a valuable tool for diagnosis that Monroe favored keeping records together as much as possible. I asked Campbell if Monroe could have the brain scan done at the hospital in Los Angeles so its results could be kept with other records already there. Campbell agreed without hesitation. My desire to keep records was sound, and so was Dr. Campbell's agreement with it. The only problem was that neither of us had any reason to suspect that those who were responsible for him in the teaching hospital might be other than honor-bright. Stupidity had occurred to me, but a cover-up had never entered my mind.

Monroe and I drove to Tarn's office for the routine visit on September 12. It proved to be anything but routine. An X-ray showed a 'spot' on Monroe's lung. Surgery was mentioned: the spot could be harmless or it could be cancerous.

I had heard that if Monroe's type of cancer spread, it would proceed almost invariably to the lung. I knew that Monroe smoked continuously. "Harmless" didn't seem likely.

An appointment for tomograms was made to determine the nature of the spot with greater accuracy.

I asked that Monroe have a brain scan the same day.

"Why do you want it?" Tarns demanded.

Why do I want it? My brain screamed and the muscles of my neck tightened and trembled. I want it because I'm worried about the way Monroe has changed and you know I'm worried! How many times must I say so? Then, realizing that I must get through to Tarns, that I couldn't become hysterical, that I had to be firm and more than emphatic, that I had to pull all the rank I could, I announced, "Because Dr. Campbell wants it... Because he thinks Monroe's problem may be neurological... Because other doctors think so, too!"

With that, Tarns capitulated and called for a brain scan.

I phoned Dr. Campbell with the news of probable lung cancer. I cancelled my upcoming appointment until I had more information. He told me to insist upon preliminary in-hospital psychiatric care for Monroe if radiation, chemotherapy, or further surgery was to be done. It seemed he hadn't completely ruled out the possibility of depression.

On September 17 I drove Monroe to the hospital and took him to the X-ray department. On the long drive to Los Angeles, I had become increasingly edgy about Tarns' casual approach to Monroe's mental condition. I knew I must make the seriousness of it so plain to Tarns that he could no longer deny it. Consequently, I left Monroe in X-ray and went to the office of the oncology group. At the desk I left a note regarding my husband. It said that by order of Dr. Campbell: "If

further radiation, chemotherapy, and/or surgery is necessary...
a psychiatrist **must** be with him **from** the beginning."

A duplicate was made. The original was delivered to
Tarns that afternoon.

My anxieties about Tarns' seeming indifference to Monroe's
mental state continued to multiply. I felt so desperate I made
an appointment to see Campbell on September 22.

As soon as I entered his office I handed him a list of
questions and concerns I had as they related to the oncology
group. I asked Campbell to get answers from Tarns to these
questions and to let him know my concerns since I had not
seemed able to get through to him. I emphasized my need to
see Tarns in his office without Monroe's being present. I did
not want Tarns to ask questions about Monroe's behavior in
the middle of a filled waiting room. I needed privacy and time
to talk with Tarns about Monroe so that I could explain my
concerns about his care.

One of the questions I wanted answered dealt with the
odds of defeating lung cancer successfully. When Campbell
obtained this answer and later relayed it to me, it was omi-
nous. Even if detected early and removed by immediate surgery, the cancer had probably already metastasized and spread
to other parts of his body, most likely to other parts of the
lung.

When we reported to Dr. Tarns' office four days later to learn
the results of the tomograms and brain scan, Monroe displayed
no great tension as to what we were to learn. I expected the
worst on both counts and did my best to cover my anxieties
in front of him.

Monroe was called into an examination room and I was
shown into a private office. Tarns met me with the news that
the tomograms revealed a tumor in the right lung which might
or might not be cancerous. He assured me that there was no

damage to Monroe's brain, that no cancer was present in the brain, but that there was "a little shrinkage" of the brain that "might account for a few of the patient's problems."

I was both elated and worried by his report. The "shrinkage" of the brain didn't frighten me because I was told it was "little." Tarns statement that there was no cancer in the brain and no damage to the brain meant to me that Monroe's mental problem was largely due to depression.

It also meant that a decision in favor of lung surgery revolved upon the advisability of extending his life for a year or so at a time when he was already despondent.

In other words, of asking him to live a little longer but with increasing mental anguish. What good, I worried, could be derived from that?

Looking at it selfishly, I thought that with in-hospital psychiatric care, Monroe's feelings toward life and toward me might improve and that we might once again find happiness in each other before he died. But the unselfish side of me saw that if Monroe was incurably despondent, he was left with nothing to look forward to but a painful death.

Given the same apparent conditions and if our roles were reversed and Monroe had to decide for me, I hoped he would say, "Let her die. Do not prolong an already ravished life through surgery that will do no good."

Then through the swirl of the battle going on in my own mind I heard the voice of Tarns saying that he would have a psychiatrist on duty two days before surgery, but that those two days wouldn't be enough time to undo all the problems the patient had developed.

I acknowledged that I didn't expect miracles and that I still didn't know about surgery. I started to explain Monroe's great personality change. I began by saying that Monroe had become so difficult to get along with...

At that instant a stocky gum-chewing figure in a white laboratory coat entered the private office without knocking.

He was the chest surgeon for the oncology group. His job was to remove cancerous lung tissue for them. From a statement he made a month later, I gathered he had overheard my complaint about Monroe.

When I demurred on surgery, the chest surgeon announced, "If she can't make up her mind, let's get out of here." His high-pressure tactic unnerved me. I had been through too much to continue calmly and reasonably. I caved in.

"As long as there is no brain damage," I capitulated, "ask Monroe." With that, the two trotted off.

Tarns returned shortly to tell me that Monroe was undecided about surgery. Tarns urged that we not delay the decision.

On the way home I exclaimed over and over to Monroe, "Isn't it wonderful that your brain isn't damaged?"

Three days later I asked Monroe if he had decided anything about surgery on his lung. I was surprised when he answered, "Yes, I want it." I didn't argue the merits of surgery with him and the possibility that the cancer had metastasized elsewhere. If his brain was not damaged, he was capable of deciding.

I asked Monroe the question one more time, a trick I had learned to make sure he was paying attention. He again said he wanted surgery.

I relayed Monroe's decision to Tarns' office immediately.

27

I visited Dr. Campbell on September 30 in a state of euphoria because Monroe's brain was not damaged. I told him that Monroe had decided on surgery and that Tarns had agreed to provide a psychiatrist two days before surgery. I babbled away that if Monroe was not brain damaged, he must be depressed. If he was depressed, maybe his depression could be cured. Maybe I had contributed to Monroe's depression by being a shrike. Maybe I had held Monroe too close to me. Campbell flattened my self-accusations by saying, "You're not a shrike." Those words made me extremely happy. They quelled a host of miserable doubts I had held against myself. Still, Monroe no longer loved me.

What had I done to lose his love? The answer meant a lot to me.

Most of the time I was rational enough to *know* that Monroe's apparent hostilities toward me were not personal. But without knowing the real cause, I could neither comprehend nor accept that his affection for me had been neutralized. I could never think of Monroe impassively. To lie nested with him, to rest my forehead between his shoulder blades, to find my worries vaporize into nothingness as Monroe's warmth enveloped me—that had been perfection.

That is why I sought so frantically and so often to bring him back to me. That is why I counted so much on the psychiatric care he would get in the hospital. Without help for him, there would be no love for me.

I knew I was no longer attractive, but I never believed that my looks would end Monroe's affection for me. I had joked that if I lost Monroe to another woman, it would be because she was smarter or funnier than I, not because she was more beautiful.

In the event that I was wrong, however, I bought a sexy caftan to dazzle Monroe. As soon as I brought it home I knew I would never wear it. Something deep inside me cautioned that the "new" Monroe would be repelled at the sight of me in the strumpety gown if he noticed me at all. I knew that my "old" Monroe would have peered at me quizzically, chuckled, and asked, "What are you made up to be?"

Dr. Campbell telephoned early in October, sounding pleased with himself for obtaining the services of a psychiatrist who would see Monroe in the hospital. I shall call the psychiatrist Lightman, a person highly esteemed by his colleagues.

A day or so later Tarns phoned. He confirmed that Lightman would visit Monroe in the hospital. He said that Lightman left the area every weekend but would see Monroe before and after surgery.

I agreed to the arrangement and assumed that other psychiatric care would be present between times, an assumption that proved to be wrong.

After what seemed an endless wait, the chest surgeon, who had been on vacation, phoned. He said that surgery was scheduled for Monday, October 20, and that Monroe was to report for hospital admittance on Sunday, October 19. Exasperated, I protested that Monroe was to be visited by a psychiatrist in the hospital for at least two days before surgery. The chest surgeon knew nothing about that plan but would investigate. He called back to say that Monroe should be at the hospital on Thursday, October 16. The psychiatrist would see Monroe that afternoon.

Hard and firm arrangements had been made at last.

28

If I could, I would omit the events which took place in the hospital between October 16 and 19, 1980, because of the kindness of the hospital's chief administrator. He listened carefully when, six months after Monroe's hospitalization, I complained about what had occurred during those days. He verified my statements and authorized restitution of Monroe's hospital expenses, almost all of which went to Monroe's insurance company and not to us. I trust also that he instituted needed reforms, for that was the main reason I went to talk with him.

A subsequent event, however, makes it necessary to begin the next phase of Monroe's story with October 16, 1980. The hospital itself is part of that story and cannot be left out.

The day began more happily than it ended. I was still torn between hopelessness over the return of Monroe's cancer and elation because Monroe would now be under psychiatric observation in the hospital and his mental health might over time be restored. As we turned into the hospital's new parking spaces, I felt a surge of affection for the hospital which I had come to know so well. In spite of fears and anxieties, Monroe and I had had fun together during his earlier stays in the building.

From the parking lot I wheeled Monroe into the cheerful lobby that led to the admissions department.

At the close of paperwork to admit Monroe, the clerk assigned him a room which I shall designate as 6-N, although that was not the actual number. Simultaneously, she handed Monroe two baggage tags with the room number on them.

"Are you sure?" I asked. "I was told it would be on a top floor."

She replied firmly that the floor was six. The number was on the baggage tag. Then Monroe was wheeled away for an "admission profile."

I proceeded to the sixth floor, thinking it might be the psychiatric section. I was eager to be in Monroe's room when Dr. Lightman arrived. I didn't know the exact time he would get there, and I didn't want us to miss the psychiatrist's first appearance.

"No Smoking, Oxygen in Use" was clearly taped across the door to room 6-N. This was obviously not the private room I had carefully arranged for. I had insisted on privacy because of Monroe's erratic behavior and in order that he could communicate freely with a psychiatrist. Monroe was a heavy smoker. He could not remain in a room where another patient depended upon the use of oxygen.

I asked for a private room. A black nurse with red hair arranged for a room in the private ward. Before taking the elevator I left word at the nurses' station on floor 6 that Monroe was to be taken to his private room as soon as he arrived. I went up to Monroe's newly assigned room to wait for him and Dr. Lightman, but the wait was long. I returned twice to the sixth floor and was told that Monroe had not yet arrived.

Around four I went to the nurses' station and asked that a search be conducted for Monroe. Shortly after that, Lightman appeared. With no patient present, Lightman had little choice but to begin Monroe's psychiatric interview with me.

We were interrupted by a nervous young nurse. She had located Monroe in a bed in room 6-N. He had been there some time, was quite settled in and not inclined to move. She said it was imperative that room arrangements be straightened out immediately.

In order to complete as much of the interview as possible in what remained of his time, Dr. Lightman and I ran down the stairs to the sixth floor. Lightman peppered me with routine questions as we went, but there was not time to offer deep confidences before we came into room 6-N in which hung a deep cloud of pipe smoke in spite of the "Oxygen in Use" sign.

As we approached Monroe's bed, I touched his foot and said, "You're supposed to be upstairs."

He replied, "I'm going to stay here. They're bringing me dinner."

Lightman asked me to leave so he could talk with Monroe. I went into the hall. On my way I passed his roommate sitting on the edge of his bed. He was complaining in broken English about the smoke in the room.

Shortly after that I saw Lightman at the nurses' station and went up to him. He said he had made contact with Monroe, that he was going to be out of town for the weekend, that he would see both of us before chest surgery on Monday. Or that is what I thought he said, although I might have misunderstood. Then he disappeared. He left without insisting to the nurses that Monroe be sent to the private room. I was sure Lightman would have insisted on a private room if he had been aware of Monroe's strange behavior.

I became numb from not knowing what to do. As a sickening panic seized me, I asked that Lightman be paged. Even as I asked, I knew it was too late, that he was no longer in the building.

I became aware of the other occupant of room 6-N. He was standing in the hall complaining to two nurses about Monroe's smoking. To solve the problem easily, I suggested that Monroe be moved immediately to the private room I had already paid for. Just then, a small, dark-haired nurse cut in, "He's promised me he won't smoke in the room. He'll go out in the hall to smoke."

"Come on," I said to Monroe, "Let's pack up and go."

"He's promised me!" the dark-hair nurse retorted harshly. "He's a grown man! He can stay here if he wants to!"

Put in my place, I wanted to scream at her, "If he were behaving like a grown man, he wouldn't be under psychiatric care. Why don't you look at his chart?" But I couldn't say that. I couldn't say anything that might push Monroe deeper into his "depression."

I was so traumatized by the nurse's flattening remark and by the destruction of my carefully prepared plans to protect Monroe and to lessen his alienation from me that I moved to a corner of a side hall. There, numbed and empty, my best efforts destroyed, my stomach pinched with pain, I leaned my clammy face into the cold wall. I could no longer think where else to go or what else to do.

Over my shoulder I heard the black nurse with red hair ask, "Do you insist that your husband be moved?"

"I insist," I sobbed; and with that Monroe was taken up to his correct room. But by then all the nerves inside me had become ignited, burned out and snapped.

I do not remember the food I had carefully ordered to please Monroe that evening. I do remember going for a walk, but I do not remember where I went. My next recollection is painfully vivid.

I found Monroe being questioned by the fidgety nurse who had earlier interrupted Dr. Lightman's interview with me. She was jotting down information about his medical history.

Still stunned by events earlier in the day, I sank into a chair near the foot of Monroe's bed. Before long I realized that most of Monroe's answers had no relation to fact. I found myself interjecting corrections. When I heard Monroe tell the nurse that he had been in the hospital only once before, I corrected his statement but I was so upset by it that I got up and went into the hall. I was tired of correcting errors. I was tired of being placed in the role of domineering wife. I was upset that Monroe might think I was condescending to him. I was shaken because something was clearly wrong and no psychiatrist was at his side to interpret his answers.

In the hall I told the fidgety nurse I absolutely had to talk to a psychiatrist or psychologist soon, that Monroe's answers were meaningless without interpretation. I begged for immediate psychiatric help for Monroe, but she said that was not possible. I found myself in an abrasive, nerve-needling argument with the nurse and nothing, absolutely nothing, was being solved.

Unremittingly routed by the events of the day, I told her I was going to leave but that psychiatric help was needed for Monroe that very night. At the elevator the argument continued. Passersby looked startled and retreated in the direction from which they had come. Sickened by my awareness that Monroe's agitated, erotic behavior had intensified with the approach of surgery and that the hospital corridors would carry his descriptive desires to a large audience, I turned my head before entering the elevator and screamed, "And whatever else you do, keep the door to his room closed!"

Nobody, apparently, honored this simple request—according to the records I later saw.

Exhausted from my beseechings that were never listened to and from the thwarting of my plans against future trauma, I fell into bed after my long drive home. I was instantly asleep.

29

By four the next morning the frustrations of the previous day shocked their way into my consciousness. The maze we had entered the day before had exits so cunningly obscured that I felt no hope of finding our way out. I lay trembling. Further sleep was out of the question, so I dressed. By daybreak I was out of the house and on my way into the mountains.

I found a firebreak and hiked to its top. In the past the mountains could be counted on to restore me; but on this Friday I no sooner got to the top of the mountain than I found myself unable to be calmed by the exertion or solaced by the clear air around me. The very stones beneath my feet called out to be trampled on, so I scrunched my way down the unstable shale of the hillside until I reached the road home.

Infuriated by my impotence in coping with a system of medical delivery that would not listen, I must have raced up and down that mountain at record speed before I managed to get home, phone Monroe's local psychiatrist, clean myself and drive to Ventura in time to talk with him before his lunch break.

He quieted me. He assured me that in a place the size of the hospital Monroe was in, he would get psychiatric care. Help would be found without my being there.

Relieved by the happy notion that the previous day was an aberration and that all my plans to help Monroe had not been blown away, I returned to Ojai and fell into a deep and healing slumber.

I have no record of the following day. Did I give up in despair? Did I sleep all that day? Did I visit Monroe? I have no recollection of that day at all.

30

On October 19, the day before Monroe was scheduled for surgery, I arrived at the hospital in mid-afternoon. Monroe was not in his room, so I asked a nurse about it. She said he had probably taken his wheelchair outside. With nothing else to do, I stood at his window and looked out. Below in the courtyard I saw Monroe, a tiny figure dressed in his best clothes, racing his wheelchair as fast as it could go across the hard-surfaced area. He had had to get there by rolling down a steep ramp. I wondered if the psychiatrist had approved of Monroe's taking his wheelchair down such a steeply graded ramp and asked about the psychiatric care Monroe had received. I learned that no psychiatrist had seen him since October 16 and that Monroe had been given the forbidden Dalmane again.

At that moment the chest surgeon put in his appearance. I told him that Monroe had been given Dalmane, that I had instructed Tarns that Monroe was never again to receive that drug. The chest surgeon promised that it would not be issued to Monroe again.

I mentioned to the surgeon my concern that Monroe should go to intensive care after surgery because there had been some problem at the time of Monroe's amputation. I had heard bells going off to sound an emergency. The surgeon replied that he was aware of the emergency and that it would not happen again.

He then said that surgery would be at 7:45 the next morning. I told him it couldn't be in the morning because the psychiatrist was to see Monroe before surgery and that I had been told surgery would be in the afternoon.

The surgeon retorted sharply that surgery would be in the morning and that was final. He turned on his heel and went out the door.

Since then I have rebuked myself for not packing Monroe's clothes and taking him home that night. I had grave doubts that lung surgery would rid him of cancer, but at the same time I was terrified that the physicians would retaliate if we walked out of the hospital and the oncology group. I did not know what other physicians I could find to help Monroe or how soon.

I was cowed by memory of my own treatment during a miscarriage. I had refused to sign an approval that the hospital could use any medication it desired. I asked to talk to my physician before signing. I was promptly carried from the hospital and left on the sidewalk to bleed until Monroe arrived to find another doctor. That was before patients had any rights at all, but it left me with no confidence in my ability to exercise whatever rights I now had.

Then, too, I knew that delay would reduce whatever chance Monroe did have for successful surgery and that he had told me he did want surgery. I was terrified that in Monroe's eyes I would become the villain.

In the hospital my fears sent me running to the stairwell that Dr. Lightman and I had raced down the previous Thursday. On the steps I let myself fall apart. A nurse came and sat beside me for a while and tried to console me. She thought I was afraid of surgery. Try as I could to explain it, nobody seemed to understand that I was terrified about not getting psychiatric care for Monroe. I had hoped Monroe would open up to a psychiatrist to alleviate whatever fears he may have had about surgery.

As I felt the minutes before Monroe's surgery slipping away without psychiatric care, I felt that all the surgeries and chemotherapies had been in vain and that nothing would ever be right again. I felt that tons of glass were crushing me. From a window at the top of the stairwell the neuropsychiatric section was in plain view. I could see the place where help could be obtained, but there was no one who would hear me. I could jump from the top of that stairwell with a note attached begging for help, but would anybody help me? Of course not. They would just scoop up my body and ignore the note, for no matter how hard or how often I had tried to get a psychiatrist to appear, no one was listening.

Even so, I could not accept the thought that help would never come. I found the head nurse and said once more that Monroe needed a psychiatrist immediately. She nodded, but no one came.

I saw the need to notify Lightman that surgery had been moved ahead to the morning. I became frantic again.

Another nurse assured me that Monroe was scheduled for surgery in the afternoon. When I confirmed the afternoon time, I saw that Monroe could still be visited by a psychiatrist before surgery if only I could reach someone. At my insistence, an attendant placed calls to the chest surgeon, to Tarns and to Lightman telling them the correct time for surgery and asking that they reach me in Monroe's room or in Ojai after ten that night. I wanted them to know that there was still time for Monroe to get psychiatric care before it was too late.

No one ever returned my call.

31

onroe's lung tumor, as I had assumed, was cancerous. When I saw Monroe on Tuesday, October 21, he was out of intensive care and in a semi-private room. I no longer objected. No psychologist had appeared or seemed likely to appear. I had been defeated on all counts and I knew it.

As I entered Monroe's room two nurses were trying to get Monroe out of bed and into a wheelchair. He managed to sit up in bed but seemed fearful of putting his remaining leg on the floor. He responded when I came in and held his hand out to me but soon returned to a dazed rocking back and forth. At the nurses' urgings, he extended his leg toward the floor and then withdrew it. A look of fear came over his face. Did he fear, I wondered, that he was about to lose his healthy leg?

Neither the nurses nor I could get him up. After a while I went to the window chairs outside his room and near the elevator to work on my needlepoint. Suddenly the elevator door opened and the chest surgeon emerged. He recognized me and said that the surgery had gone well and Monroe would recover soon. The median lobe of his right lung had been removed, the doctor added, and they were quite sure the sarcoma had spread from the original source.

The surgeon paused to let his message sink in. Then he suggested that a new type of chemotherapy had been developed that might be used. My look at him must have told him that I thought his suggestion was not only hopeless but unprofessional—when laid against the history of unsuccessful lung cancer recoveries. At any rate, I said nothing and he changed the subject. He volunteered that he and the psychiatrist had decided that Monroe didn't need a psychiatrist before surgery. Then he added gratuitously, that he didn't know *"how I was going to get along with the guy once you get him home."* He turned and walked away.

Stunned by the callousness of his remark, I stared at his retreating back in disbelief. In a marriage that had been extraordinarily happy during most of its forty years, he had recalled the one phrase he overheard when he barged into the private conversation between Dr. Tarns and me, just as I had begun to detail Monroe's personality change.

God bless you for your sweet compassion, I thought bitterly as the surgeon rounded a corner and disappeared into another corridor. I wondered if he had bothered to tell the psychiatrist how desperately I had called for help.

The next afternoon, October 22, I found Monroe looking well but groggy. He was watching cartoons on a tiny television set held by a long arm over his bed. He was not interested in my presence, so I stepped into the hall. No sooner did I get into the hall than I was accosted by the dark-haired nurse who had put me down prior to Monroe's surgery. "Does your husband always act like that? I've got to know if that's the way he always acts!"

I retorted, "I don't know what you mean by 'how he acts.' I just got here." I felt my voice begin to rise. "Why ask me? Ask the psychiatrist who was supposed to see him! Ask a psychiatrist if you can find one around this place..."

With that the tall figure of Dr. Lightman danced his way toward me. He was glancing at room numbers as he passed each door. At the height of my angry encounter with the nurse, Lightman caught sight of me and came forward.

"Here's the psychiatrist now," I told the nurse. Still ruffled, I demanded, "Ask him. He ought to know how my husbands acts!" With that, the nurse vanished down the corridor.

To Lightman's polite "How are you?" I retorted that I was in a rage. He didn't ask why but asked if I knew anything about a brain scan done on my husband in September.

"Of course," I replied, suddenly brought to attention. "Who called for it?"

"I did. And Dr. Campbell did. And Dr. Lorraine did."

"Who is this Dr. Lorraine?"

I replied that she was a psychologist who said "neurology must be ruled out" before anything else was done, and she had been the one who referred Monroe to Campbell. And while I was answering Lightman's question, I realized with painful intuition what I had hoped could not be so: that neurology was involved and that Monroe's brain was damaged, and I heard myself gasp, "But it all makes more sense!"

Lightman looked at me sharply and briefly and said, "Let's go in and take a look at him."

Monroe was in bed, his head and torso elevated. He was still watching television. Lightman asked him several questions. Monroe diverted his gaze briefly from the cartoons to reply, but his interest in Lightman soon disappeared and his eyes went back to his cartoon friends.

When Lightman and I were once again in the corridor, he expressed his opinion that Monroe's brain was severely impaired, but he wanted to confirm his tentative diagnosis. He arranged to meet me at his office the next morning. As he scribbled his address and phone number, I noticed his distinctive handwriting. It was strangely sinuous. He told me to telephone him if I needed help before I visited him. I think now that he would have helped us earlier if he had been told before the surgery about the brain scan.

I looked forward to seeing Lightman again. Much of my encounter with him on the previous day was printed indelibly on my brain, not only for what was said but for what was not said. By now Lightman might know more because he would have seen the scan of Monroe's brain. He might be able to help me understand.

I desperately wanted to understand.

But even as I looked forward to a discussion with this man whose mind was razor sharp, I reminded myself to be wary. I had perceived that he was skilled enough and intelligent enough to recognize a serious problem once he encountered it. But I also reminded myself that he had not put in an appearance on Monday morning nor had he telephoned me. I did not know why he had failed to do so and I was aware that I might have been wrong about his intention to visit Monroe before surgery. Nevertheless, I was prepared to find him defensive not only on his own behalf but as to why Tarns had told me that Monroe's brain was not damaged even though records to the contrary had been in his possession for some time. I was determined to remain on guard, but I was equally determined to hear Lightman out.

Lightman's office was not far from the hospital. Facing me as I entered his room was a long, dark tuxedo type couch, the kind whose pillows squash down with the weight of one's body, the sort of couch it's fun to bounce up and down on. I longed to bounce, but restrained myself. Nonetheless, the couch made me feel jolly and able to handle myself without bursting into tears.

Lightman wasted no time in telling me that the frontal lobes of Monroe's brain were indeed severely damaged. Then he offered an explanation for Tarns' mis-statement to me regarding the brain scan: That Tarns had understood the brain scan was to determine if the cancer had spread to the brain. He hadn't understood that I was interested in other kinds of damage to the brain.

"The compartmentalization of modern medicine!" I suggested in an attempt not to be too disagreeable. But I found Tarns' explanation utterly fatuous. I doubted that Lightman himself could believe it.

Lightman made no effort to explain why he had not appeared on Monday. He seemed to feel no need to defend himself. For that I gave him a plus.

In answer to Lightman's question, "When did you first notice anything wrong with your husband," I cited Monroe's recovery from the first chemotherapy, which seemed slow and to the "bad Methotrexate" of August, 1977, the time when the granular tissue which had been growing steadily across the exposed bone practically disintegrated in front of our eyes. After that, Monroe had appeared withdrawn. (Though I didn't know it at the time of my consultation with Lightman, nor had I even thought about it, the hospital could no longer be sued over the bad Methotrexate. The length of time allowed by the Statute of Limitations had run out.)

But when I became seriously troubled by the change in Monroe was right after the emergency had developed following the amputation. There had been a nurses' "scramble." After that, I explained, Monroe had behaved very differently than before.

Lightman brusquely turned aside my discussion of this episode. At the time I wondered why. Perhaps he thought the discussion fruitless. Perhaps he thought it was no time for one physician to express shock at what had happened in the hospital following the work of other professionals and/or its significance. (At the time the Statute of Limitations had not run out, although it would not be long before it did, as I later found out.)

Lightman asked if I would accept more surgery for Monroe when the cancer returned. With that statement he reminded me not only that the cancer would return but that I would have to face it and make a decision about it.

I know that before the lung surgery, I would have preferred death for a brain-damaged Monroe rather than prolonging his life, but would I have actually agreed if the decision had been mine to make? I told Lightman honestly that I didn't know what I might do but that I knew how I would choose for myself and that I had put in writing my wishes against the use of heroic measures to keep me alive. Lightman appeared to smile approval of my action.

"What will you do when Monroe dies?" Lightman demanded. He stressed the word "dies," perhaps to test if I really understood what lay ahead for Monroe and me. He asked if I would move near my son. He seemed to be trying to find out how dependent I was on others for moral support. I found myself saying that I was far and away the youngest of my siblings, that I still had to take care of my mother and that I didn't believe in moving in with my son. Again, I thought he smiled approval of my independence.

He emphasized that dealing with a sick person was extremely difficult, that people develop all sorts of hostile feelings when they spend a lot of time with the sick. I acknowledged past feelings of savagery. I don't remember if I told him I had passed beyond that phase. I know I felt secure within myself that I would never return to those unreasonable rages against Monroe because I knew he was not at fault for doing what had formerly enraged me.

Then Lightman said something about Monroe's lack of awareness of what was going on around him. He said Monroe looked unhappy, but was not necessarily unhappy. He said something about a convalescent hospital. He was telling me that I need feel no guilt if I had Monroe institutionalized.

Suddenly, Monroe's recent treatment in the hospital and the snickering final comment of the chest surgeon streaked through my brain and I blurted to Lightman, "I don't want anybody to laugh at him!" And then I felt myself screaming, "And I don't want anybody to feel sorry for me either..." I looked away to stop my tears and tried to explain my outrage by adding, "No woman ever had a better husband than I."

But before I spoke that truth, the memory of another man whose brain had snapped came crashing through my own brain, and I heard an old fool saying to my mother, "My dear, I don't know why you put up with him," and I wanted to kill the old gossip and to kill my mother for even listening, for what right had she to listen to such words about the gentle man who had loved her for sixty-five years and had only become intractable at the age of eighty-nine?

I realize that what I have written seems to throw a shadow over Dr. Lightman and the help he gave me. If this is so, it reflects my own state of mind at the time of the consultation and the need to compress the contents of our discussion. In actuality, the help I received from him far outweighed my cynicism about his loyalty to his hospital and the doctors associated with it. It was he who told the truth about Monroe. With that truth to help me, I was able to prepare myself for the future.

His telling me that Monroe was not responsible for his anti-social behavior lightened my load. And most wonderful of all, he had assured me that the damage to Monroe's brain had left him unable to feel pain as intensely as normal people would. Death, as it took him, would not hurt him too much.

At the door Lightman extended his hand. I hesitated before taking it, not because of any reservation I had, but because I noticed the articulation of his little finger with its carpal bone skewed inward. Monroe's college roommate had had the same anomaly. (I almost raised Lightman's hand to inspect it closely but decided not to. He could have forgotten my mentioning that I had studied physical anthropology and thought I had really gone over the edge.)

Instead, I grasped his hand and went on my way knowing that the husband I had loved was already dead and never would return.

In the hospital lay a child in Monroe's body, a child who would not live long and who might still need me if only to help him die.

32

Had I not spent that hour with Dr. Lightman in his office I do not know if I could have borne the coming days. Perhaps, too, the very numbness that I felt helped me to endure. Of this I am sure: The time spent with Lightman had much to do with the direction of our coming lives. So, too, did the hospital and its attending physicians, but for different reasons. As Lightman's questions and explanations helped me select a path, the mistreatment of Monroe in the hospital steeled me to follow a course that would once have seemed impossible but from which, once the decision was made, I never turned aside. Whenever doubts began to weaken me or my confidence began to flag, the specter of the hospital came back to keep me on our course.

The last days of Monroe's stay in the hospital were grim or grimly-comic, with one episode that lightened my day and eased the road Monroe and I would take. It occurred when a tall woman, a psychologist who was pretty in her sloppy rainwear, stopped to talk with me in the hospital corridor. She had come at Lightman's behest from conducting a series of tests that measured the functionings of Monroe's brain. She chatted about Monroe and me as comfortably as if she and I were old friends pulling weeds from our gardens.

I lamented that Monroe looked upon me as a chambermaid.

"That is what can be expected," she responded. With Monroe's type of brain dysfunction he would never again have feelings of love toward me, his son, or anyone else. She volunteered that lots of women leave their husbands forever when this happens.

I confided that I had left Monroe once, but added, "I sent him a present every day."

"You're a real nice lady," she commented in a voice that was genuine and warm. Instantly, any remaining guilt I felt was dissipated. She had driven it away without even the wave of a wand.

The woman's testing had confirmed the diagnosis of frontal lobe dysfunction. I telephoned this information to Jeff and Mike. As I explained the diagnosis, I could almost hear weights fall from their shoulders. They understood now that Monroe's indifference to them was in no way personal, that the frontal lobes of his brain had been damaged so severely that he was no longer capable of returning their love.

The truth, I found, was easy to relate. The truth helped each of us feel whole again.

Before leaving the hospital that Friday I took pains to insure that Monroe would not be discharged the next day; but when I got to the hospital on Saturday, I learned that Monroe was discharged and ready to go home.

I couldn't believe it.

I protested to the resident sitting at the nurses' station.

I told the resident I couldn't handle the situation. I had not hired help. If two nurses had trouble getting Monroe out of bed, how could I manage alone?

The resident indicated that other people manage.

At that moment the spidery handwriting of Dr. Lightman on the chart in front of the young physician sprang into my view. I did not know what Lightman had written, but I took a gamble.

"Read what the psychiatrist wrote!" I pointed my finger toward Lightman's writing. "This is no ordinary case!"

The resident grunted an "oh" after reading it, then shrugged his shoulders. The discharge papers, he reiterated, were already signed.

I felt my arms stiffen and my knuckles tighten against the counter's edge. I could contain myself no longer.

"I won't take him home today! I can't take him home today! I'll take him home tomorrow!"

As I began to run to the elevator I heard the black nurse with the red hair say softly, "You have that right."

When I came back for Monroe the next morning, his bags were packed. He was in a wheelchair wearing his pale blue blazer. It complemented his graying hair. He looked elegant and distinguished. It was hard to realize that inwardly he had changed so much.

At the nurses' station I picked up the medications he would need at home. In the packet was a bottle of the forbidden Dalmane. I didn't protest. I no longer felt surprise that it had been issued over my repeated objections. I simply left it in the package and I have it still.

Behind the desk two residents were arguing about the time to remove the staples that clinched Monroe's incision. They agreed, finally, to leave the staples in place until Monroe returned to the oncology group the next month. With that decision made, I turned Monroe in his wheelchair to face the elevator while awaiting the last item from pharmacy.

At that moment a Dr. Akin approached the elevator with a train of interns behind him. I recognized him as the resident who had worked in the cancer ward during Monroe's first admission. He was now a teaching physician.

"You don't remember us..." I began as the elevator reserved for staff stopped at our floor.

"Oh, yes, I do," he responded after glancing at Monroe. Dr. Akin then entered the elevator and, as he and the interns shifted to face forward, he nodded in Monroe's direction.

"He's the dean of the School of Opthal..." Before he could finish his sentence, the elevator door slid shut. The eyebrows of the two residents who had argued the time to remove Monroe's staples shot up in marked surprise at the deference given Monroe. They almost saluted as they heard Akin's parting sentence.

Without saying a word, they simultaneously rose, turned Monroe's wheelchair around, wheeled him out of the corridor, took off his coat and shirt and removed the staples and dressed him again. Bowing, almost kowtowing, they sent us on our way.

It was funny. It was shockingly elitist and revealing. Two vastly different modes of medicine practiced in the same hospital. It was as if we were in India again: Brahmin/ Untouchable; sterile hypodermic needles for the upper castes, already used ones for the lower castes.

While driving Monroe home, a great wave of tender admiration came over me. He had always insisted that the same amount of time be scheduled for charity patients as for anyone else. All of his patients, he made clear, were human beings deserving of the best care.

33

I felt so beaten at the end of Monroe's hospital stay that I made an appointment to see psychiatrist Campbell again. I remember nothing about that visit except grieving over and over, again and again, "They never heard a word I said..."

But had they heard?

After going over old notes and records, both the hospital's and mine, my thinking has changed. Some, I believe, heard nothing; some heard what their specialities had compartmentalized them to hear. One, I believe, heard but diverted my attempts to find the truth. He had his own reasons, I think, not to acknowledge my pleas.

Though I became debilitated by despondency after bringing Monroe home from the hospital, my torpor did not last long. There were causes for this.

I had already assumed responsibility for the financial and physical comforts of Monroe and me. I knew that if I didn't carry on, no one else would.

I had been given insight into Monroe's difficulties. I no longer expected more from him than he was able to fulfill. I became relaxed in my efforts to help him. I did not feel hurt and tormented as I had before. A deep hole still remained because of the loss of the friendship Monroe could no longer give me, but I stopped blaming myself for losing his love. I stopped burdening myself with fruitless efforts to regain it.

Once I understood the cause of Monroe's behavior, I could accept it. I could explain it to friends. I could explain it to visitors before they entered the house so that they, too, could accept it. And it was nice to have visitors again.

Though insight and independence were fundamental to my recovery, it was two tiny incidents that shook me out of lethargy and flexed my claws for fight. These came in the form of communications from the hospital. On the surface they were innocuous enough. It was largely what they failed to say that stung me into action.

The first communication was a hospital bill several pages long. It was a copy of a statement to be paid almost entirely by our insurance company. In spite of the fact that payment of the bill was not up to us, I studied it carefully. There was one, and only one, item listed for the three-day period between Monroe's admission to the hospital and the day before surgery. These were the three days when Monroe should have received psychiatric care but didn't. They were days when we would both have been better off if we had stayed at home but were told to be there. During those three days Monroe had been issued one pair of hospital stockings. For this "care," the tab was almost one thousand dollars, a huge sum in those days.

I protested Monroe's treatment to the insurance company and sent a copy of my letter to several people. Some six weeks later, shortly before Christmas, 1980, I received a response from the Dean of the University's School of Medicine. He had talked with the oncologists involved and had composed a carefully worded, conciliatory letter in which he shared "their explanation" with me. "Their explanation" justified the four-day preoperative admission with "...there was some doubt as to the extent of the preoperative counseling or therapy that would be required..."

Their explanation infuriated me. If there was some doubt, why did Monroe spend any extra days at all in the hospital?

Why did they doubt? Our Ventura psychiatrist had insisted on a psychiatrist in attendance from the beginning. That message had been relayed by me in writing to Tarns. He had agreed to it. What was the doubt?

If there was doubt, why was it never transmitted to me?

Doctors Campbell and Lorraine had insisted upon a scan of Monroe's brain a month before surgery. Why had Dr. Lightman not been told before surgery that a brain scan existed? I felt damn sure Dr. Tarns had never given that piece of information to the Dean of the Medical School. Why hadn't he?

I took the dean's letter in both my hands to tear it into shreds, but I threw it instead onto the growing pile of papers relating to Monroe's illness. Their explanation is so damn shallow, I raged to myself, *It's nothing but a sink full of mud!*

Not until months later did I learn how terribly turbid it was.

34

Writing and the seclusion of my little room grew more essential to me daily. I could retreat there in my rages and transfer my fury to my pen or to my typewriter keys. I could no longer express my frustrations to Monroe, but I could defuse them within my little room. It was there I tried to write things out, to reduce my grievances against the hospital staff and its cavalier treatment of Monroe. It was there I could weep with no one to see.

Each night I would go into the quiet of my room and jot down the simple events of the day, of my walks in the morning before Monroe woke up, of the singing of the birds, of my recollections of Monroe and the family before he got sick.

Most of these efforts I tossed out the next day, but in clearing up my desk recently I have come across some of those essays. I have been amazed to find how many open with the dreary, "I am so lonely...," but I have been equally amazed to find that before I had finished a page my spirits, more often than not, had begun to soar. In many of those little compositions I was with Monroe again, walking and laughing and talking things over.

I realize now that in the seclusion of my little room in the year before Monroe died I had already found him again.

By the spring of 1981 I was writing regularly, rarely ending a day without transferring my thoughts to paper. After I had emptied my brain of sorrows and joys and grievances, I would fall into immediate, untroubled sleep.

Sometimes when I was typing, Monroe asked what I was writing. I told him I was writing about him and the people we knew. If Monroe said he would like to hear what I had written, I chose a happy story about family or about him and his work. Sometimes I read anecdotes: of the time he shoved aside his other work to drive an artist with a detached retina to a neighboring city for immediate surgical care; of the times he whipped out his checkbook on behalf of an impoverished student; of the time he returned from a convention and reported, "We must be getting old. The guys don't talk about sex any more. They just complain about their hemorrhoids!"

I read to him of the time he had become director of clinics at the optometry school in Berkeley in 1969. With two partners in his Ojai office he could leave for days at a stretch to be in Berkeley. Almost as soon as he took over the job, he found that the optometry school had fallen behind financially. This seemed incredible to Monroe because charges by the school for lenses and frames were on a level with private practitioners.

Breakage by student learners was blamed, but Monroe doubted there was that much breakage. He had a quick check made on invoices from the laboratories that supplied uncut lenses to the university. Monroe noticed that the school, item for item, paid more than he paid in private practice. That was strange because purchases in large quantities are usually charged less, not more, than purchases made of smaller quantities.

Monroe asked an assistant to survey invoices from all laboratories. The assistant reported that though the lenses had been put to bid, estimates from all the laboratories were almost identical.

Monroe invited representatives from all the local laboratories to the school. He showed the results of the telltale survey. He told them he couldn't prove collusion but that they would get no more laboratory work from the university until they turned in honest bids.

The next day a representative telephoned, admitted guilt, and asked for another chance. With one laboratory capitulating, the others followed. Not surprisingly, the clinic was out of the red by the following year.

Sometimes Monroe laughed when I read to him; sometimes he smiled. I think he liked to have me write about his life.

Not long after we were home again in Ojai I realized that the shock from further surgery had reduced Monroe's comprehension below its previous level. His incontinence of urine, his increased apathy and indecisiveness were not due, I realized, to the drugs administered in the hospital because he was no longer taking medication.

Perhaps it didn't matter any more. Monroe would not have long to live and he was less restless now. He seemed to stop striving for something he could not attain. I did not know it at that time, but before long a great tranquility would grow between Monroe and me. Not all the change was in Monroe. It was also in me.

In the quiet of my little room I wondered how to get the transgressions of the health care practitioners recognized by them so that no similar mistreatment would happen to others. During Monroe's hospitalization I had seen the staff set examples for the student nurses and interns that were barbarously unworthy of any teaching institution.

I tried to think what Monroe would have done, how he would have gotten the hospital and staff to make improvements.

I thought of legal action and wondered why there were so many malpractice suits. I thought of Monroe at the School of Optometry in Berkeley. While he was dean, only one malpractice suit had been brought against his department. Was it because errors had never been made? Was it because the patient knew what to expect because it had been explained to him? Or was it because the staff were trained to listen and cared enough to correct their errors and to admit to them if errors had been made?

I remembered how Monroe's door had been open so he could hear complaints from patients, faculty, and students. He even heard complaints from mothers, outraged because an offspring had failed to make entrance requirements. He often came home exhausted from listening to grievances, but he took them seriously. He took them as part of his job. Maybe that was why lawsuits had not developed.

Monroe had listened.

Perhaps the chief administrator of the hospital would listen to my concerns, especially about Monroe's three days in the hospital when nothing was done.

I decided to see him in person. I knew I must have my statement of the problem and my evidence in perfect order so that I could convince him in a short time that my complaints were valid.

My request for an audience was granted in March. By the end of the thirty-minute interview I had told the events of Monroe's pre-operative hospitalization and had expressed my deep grievances against one physician in particular. The administrator listened attentively but said he needed to investigate.

Not many days later he wrote that my "concerns and position are supported by our records." He cancelled all hospital charges for the first three days and returned the money to the insurance company.

In a later letter he said he could not respond directly to the concerns I had about the doctors involved but had sent copies of all correspondence to their attention.

Cheered by the belief that I was making some impact on the great bureaucracy behind the hospital's walls, I wrote the surgeon in charge of the oncology group. He was the one who had done Monroe's first surgery. I had already decided that there was no sense in facing Dr. Tarns with my accusations. He had not listened before. There was no reason to expect him to pay attention now.

I asked the head of the oncology group for time to present evidence to him of malfeasance within his group. To assure him of my reliability I reminded him of the correspondence forwarded to him by the chief administrator. The date of my letter was May 7, 1981.

35

I knew after Monroe's chest surgery that I could not avoid a decision about Monroe's future care. Any oncologist who attended him in the future must not only be competent, but compassionate enough to let Monroe die once the cancer again took hold. He must not intervene to keep Monroe alive. He must intervene only to alleviate pain.

I reached that decision in the refuge of my little room. I reached it because I knew that however much I had depended on Monroe to provide meaning to my life, I must not extend his life to serve me as a crutch.

To reach that decision about another's life is not easy. It is still less easy to hold firm when the possibility of retreat is about to end.

Monroe had been instructed to come in for further X-rays in March, 1981, to determine whether the cancer had spread again. I knew that if I didn't take Monroe in for X-rays, I would have, in fact, made the decision to let Monroe die if his cancer had once again presented itself. March, therefore, was the month beyond which we could not turn back. I found I could not struggle through that anxious time alone. I could not face the day Monroe might look at me accusingly and ask me, why? Why had I not taken him to be X-rayed? Why had I not allowed his life to be extended a few more weeks by one more surgery.

I had always told everything to Monroe. I could no longer keep my worry from him.

During a drive, I parked the car upon a bluff overlooking Lake Casitas. I asked Monroe if he knew that the cancer which had been removed from his lung had spread from its original source. He said he knew. I explained I had not taken him to be X-rayed because, even if the picture showed cancer, there wasn't much that could be done. There could be only so many surgeries and if the cancer metasticizes again and surgery done, other cancer cells would reproduce elsewhere.

I told him that if he were to die from lung cancer, he would feel little pain. I asked him how he felt about not going to a doctor for more X-rays.

"About the same as you," he responded.

From the time of his amputation, conversation between us had been largely a soliloquy. This day was no different. When I asked him if I had made him unhappy by talking about his possible death, he said, "No."

I started the car again and began to sing. Monroe joined me immediately. "You are my sunshine, my only sunshine," we caroled as we drove the highway, two old crows, neither of us able to carry a tune. I do not know what Monroe was really feeling. I, for one, was singing my fears away.

I shall never know how much Monroe understood about what I said to him that day, but I believe he understood me every bit as much as he understood the surgeons who urged lung surgery. I believe it would have been equally easy to talk Monroe out of a needless surgery as it was to talk him into it.

Monroe agreed immediately to my proposal; it had taken him three days to agree to theirs.

Then it occurred to me, why an oncologist at all? An oncologist, eventually, would send Monroe to a hospital if only to die there. Hospital personnel would make every effort to prolong Monroe's life. That is their discipline. But they wouldn't take him for drives in the afternoon, and they wouldn't ply him with delicacies that would make him happy though possibly shorten his life, and they wouldn't wheel him along the promenade at the beach and they wouldn't take him picnicking in the woods.

Realizing that, the solution became simple. Monroe would stay at home until he died. I would allow no one to intervene until Monroe's pain became acute and then only with medicine to relieve the hurt.

I asked our family physician if he would cooperate. He agreed with such ease that I realized Monroe and I were far from the first to turn our backs on a medical code so archaic that it could not accept death as a release from life.

During the summer that followed, Monroe began to lose weight steadily, a sign that the cancer had returned; but he saw no physician and had no X-rays because that was the way we had planned it. By that time, even had we wanted to turn back, it was too late.

36

Early in June, 1981, I sat at my desk opening my correspondence. An envelope from the hospital caught my eye. I tore it open, hoping it was from the chief of oncology, the man to whom I had written in the expectation that he would give me a time in which to explain my concerns. What I found instead was a letter signed by an employee who stated that the chief of oncology was "...unavailable for a meeting at this time..." and that I should respond by "stating the specific details of the grievances you alledged (sic) to in your letter."

I began to laugh, not joyfully, I must admit. I had never expected to be thought addle-pated enough to receive the "go-climb-a-glass-hill" letter. I had first heard of such a diversionary tactic when I was a tiny child in my parent's home at a small dinner party. A heavy-set broker had been seated across the table from me. As his jowls waggled from side to side, I heard him announce that he would get rid of the crazy old lady who was dissatisfied with his services. He would ask her to detail her specific grievances in writing. I must have shown my bewilderment as to why he wanted the crazy old lady to do that, for my father leaned over to me and said, "It's like that fairy tale I read to you... Where the king protected his throne by giving an impossible task to his daughter's suitors... He demanded they climb a glass hill... My friend is sure the old lady can't possibly put all of her complaints together on paper... It's too hard... It's like asking her to climb a mountain made of slippery glass."

Now, at age sixty-four, I was the old woman who had been told to "go climb a glass hill;" but was I crazy as well? Had I not written a reasonable letter? Had I not had good references? Had I not gathered my evidence and presented it convincingly to the chief administrator?

I tossed the letter onto the stack of medical records on my desk. It landed on top of the looseleaf binder in which I had carefully summarized my grievances. I had included a tight chronology of events, color-coding each item to match the documents appended at the end. I had known the chief surgeon's time was valuable and I had organized carefully to prevent the waste of it.

My eyes turned from my scrupulously arranged medical notebook and wandered to the miscellany of little stories and essays I had found comfort in writing. I looked again at the stack of medical notes and saw my right hand drawing them towards me. Then my left hand began to pull my heap of personal jottings forward. As they approached each other, their contents began to coalesce within my brain, their information dovetailing into one case history, far more loving and revealing than hard facts by themselves.

I would write Monroe's story, perhaps for my eyes alone, and I would weed out more facts to show that what I wrote was true. Then, too, if what I wrote proved good enough perhaps someplace, somewhere, sometime, I could convince some key influential people that dreadful medical errors could be avoided if medics would learn to listen. Maybe then they would do something about it.

But should I try to climb the slippery peak the oncology group was counting on to thwart me? I doubted it. There would be no helping hands to get me to the top, only more and more obstructions to keep me down.

37

I moved to obtain more facts. Having fixed the radical change in Monroe's behavior at the time his leg was amputated, I asked the hospital for information about what had occurred at that time. In September, 1981, I received an operation report and discharge summary from the hospital. One sentence jumped out at me from the page:

> *Postoperatively the patient was given a dose of Demerol on the ward and promptly developed Cheyne-Stokes respiration, became cyanotic and was in marked respiratory distress.*

Monroe couldn't breathe following a dose of Demerol! He had turned blue from lack of oxygen. Something, indeed, had happened!

But a summary is not proof, I was told. That could be found only in the daily notes of the hospital's staff. It took me eleven more months to obtain these notes, largely because of my preoccupation with Monroe and my own decline in energy and ability to resolve problems. Then it took me another two days to muster courage to read them. When I did, I learned that at 15:25 (3:25pm) Monroe was checked out of surgery. He was in a reactive, responsive condition, with good color. Twenty minutes later he was in a private room, not a recovery room, and was "sleeping, not arousing to verbal stimuli."

Though a doctor's order clearly stated "No Demerol until 2000," a nurse gave it to Monroe at 1700 hours—three hours ahead of schedule. Fifteen minutes later a nurse found Monroe breathing laboriously, "using accessory muscles." His facial skin was "dusky—or cyanotic." He didn't respond to verbal stimuli. Another fifteen minutes passed before a doctor administered an antidote to Demerol. That was at the time, I am sure, that I heard a man yell, "God damn it. I told you not to do that!"

Two hours later Monroe was again found with respiratory distress "as described earlier." Thirty minutes later, after more antidote had been given, Monroe appeared to be better, according to the daily notes of hospital staff.

When I carefully inspected the anesthesia records, I noticed that Monroe also received 200 mg. Demerol in surgery. There is no indication in the record that the Demerol had been reversed by any antidote whatever.

It is no wonder that Monroe could not breathe, that his lungs could not supply his brain with the oxygen they needed to keep him healthy.

Physician's Desk Reference, 1996, page 2023, includes the following: "Serious overdosage with meperdine (Demerol) is characterized by respiratory depression, Cheyne-Stokes respiration, cyanosis, extreme somnolence..." It notes that death may follow.

Demerol is extremely toxic.

The description of the emergency has left no doubt in my mind that by the time Monroe was revived on February 3, 1978, his ability to reason and to judge and to love was gone forever. But because Monroe had seemed withdrawn before the amputation, I cannot prove a problem did not exist before that time. A brain can be affected by a bad combination of chemicals, such as the "bad" Methotrexate Monroe had been given earlier. Toxins produced by the cancer itself have been said to cause symptoms Monroe displayed, known as Pick's frontal lobe syndrome. (There is, it should be added, no known history of an inherited malady called Pick's Disease among Monroe's ancestors or relatives.) But, whatever else may have contributed to the problem, of this I am convinced: The cyanotic episode precipitated or caused severe behavioral changes. The difference in Monroe's personality and behavior before and after the event was too sharp to be otherwise.

Staff notes from the hospital at the time of the amputation reveal questions and suggestions about Monroe's mental state. They crop up repeatedly in entries by nurses, physicians, and physical therapists. They indicate neurological problems and doubts that depression alone was involved. No one ever told me about these concerns even though I myself had raised them. Why was I never told? Was there a reason not to tell me?

I had assumed all along that Monroe's leg had been removed by an orthopedic surgeon. The operation report showed that Tarns himself was surgeon in charge of the amputation.

With sickening thought I realized that there was no way Tarns could not have known about the traumatic episode following surgery. There was no way he could not have recognized the possibility of its brain-damaging effects. If he denied this, even to himself, he could not deny that he was "notified of the patient's condition" when he came to Monroe's room on the day after surgery.

With bitter awareness, I came to believe that the one doctor to whom I had steadily appealed for help in getting psychological care for Monroe was the same man who would never, never encourage it. I tried to tell myself that he might not have taken me seriously when I first asked for help, but how could he not have begun to wonder when I asked so often about Monroe's mental health and possible brain damage? How could he not have been reminded when experts demanded a brain scan? Didn't that **mean** something to him? And how could he not have been reminded when the report on the brain scan done in September, 1980, noted affective changes and stated in capital letters, "FRONTAL LOBE ATROPHY, MARKED?"

Did Tarns have no responsibility to tell me this?

Never once did Tarns hint to me of the hideous episode that triggered the respiratory distress. Never once did he emphasize the heavy odds against chest surgery successfully ridding Monroe of cancer. Never once did he try to talk us out of the final surgery. Instead, he encouraged it. He left Monroe and me in a forest of nettles and thorns to work our way out without help or guidance (as his corporation pocketed the profits.)

Among some physicians, it is said, there is an unwritten commandment, never to be broken: Thou shalt not reveal the errors of thy colleagues, for ours is the kingdom of heaven and to do so would tarnish our godly image.

38

One day after I had received the psychometric report we were visited by a friend who is a psychiatrist. "You should put Monroe in a convalescent hospital," he volunteered after reading the report, "he'll never know the difference."

"He may not know the difference," I replied with conviction, "but I will."

I had spent too much time with my father, brother and mother in convalescent hospitals during the previous twelve years not to know the difference; not to know the hopeless, vacant forlornness on the faces inside; not to know what is done to and for them in the name of medicine.

My mother was "saved" from death by pneumonia three times when she was almost a hundred. She could move one finger to scratch her nose and she could suck food from the syringe I inserted into her mouth. She did not know me and she could not see me. She was too deaf to hear the ancient woman screeching and howling in the bed beside her, her muscles contracting in tetanus-like display. The woman was quiescent only when she was feverish or heavily sedated. Often the sedatives were not strong enough to stop her screams. One day she was feverish and nurses were put on constant watch. They did not let her die. It was against the rules to do so. Three days later she was screeching and contorting as wildly as she did before.

My father's heart stopped when he was ninety-one years old, but the hospital's efficient nurse pounded his heart and started it beating again. By her disciplined professional act she extended my father's life three months. By a thump on his heart she brought back to life a man who wanted to die, who recognized that his brains were gone and who had often said that his life, now useless, was no life at all.

I had no intention of letting these things happen to the man I loved.

I do not advocate keeping all the aged and dying at home. It must be an individual decision. If I had been ten years older, I might not have had the strength to do it. If I had had to go out to earn a living, I could not have done it. If it had not been paramount to me that no one would ever again intervene to extend the existence that was Monroe's life, I might not have held firm.

It was, however, paramount to me. I did weaken. I did have terrible anxieties about my decision, but I never gave in.

Mike moved a hospital bed into the living room in September, 1981, because Monroe could no longer negotiate the steps down to his bed in the library.

Monroe found the wheelchair easier to use than his canes. With a wheelchair he could move from his overstuffed chair to his bed without encountering extreme changes in elevation. He needed less help from me in lifting or lowering himself.

I built a ramp from the front porch to the driveway so we could continue our rides in the car and our walks with the wheelchair.

Ten days before Christmas our family physician wrote Monroe's first prescription against pain—Emperin with codeine. Monroe took five tablets only between that day and the day he died.

A few days before Christmas, Jeff and Francia brought their five and six-year-old boys to spend the holidays with us. From Monroe's bed in the living room he could see across the garden to the bridle path and the street, and he could look down into his library. He watched with seeming enjoyment as his grandchildren decorated the evergreen tree I had placed there.

The little boys buzzed with excitement. It was the first time they had trimmed a tree. They concentrated on the lower branches while their father took care of the higher ones. After hanging an ornament in a new place, we heard first one child and then the other whisper, "This ornament looks 'lonesome'." Then they proceeded to surround the "lonesome" decoration with other ornaments. Between the bunched ornaments were enormous gaps. The result was sensational. It was the prettiest tree we ever had.

Before New Year's we went to the picnic grounds at Rose Valley. A nippy breeze was blowing, but the sky was blue and sparkling. Monroe was so eager to participate that he hopped with little help from the car to the picnic table, where he sat while the boys engaged him in a game of "keep-away." Jeff had to carry his father back to the car.

A month later I was awakened in the middle of the night by Monroe's voice in steady speech. I found him sitting in his easy chair. He was reading from the Sierra Club's magazine about camping equipment. He didn't make a mistake although many of the words were complicated. Was he remembering happier days gone by? I hope so.

Two days after that Monroe tipped off a stool while I was trying to hold him. He rolled onto the carpet. He looked surprised for a second and then beautifully calm. I fetched a mirror and held it to his lips. There was no mist of life, and so I phoned the doctor knowing neither he nor anyone else could prolong Monroe's existence again.

There is no calm like the calm that comes with the death of one who has endured too long. I cried, of course; but I did not cry in sorrow. My tears were like the tears at a wedding, caused by a kaleidoscope of happy memories.

I refused company that night. I didn't want anyone to try to comfort me, for I was already comforted.

The next morning when I began my walk, a fulsome moon still shimmered in a light blue sky. I was not alone, and I knew it, for pale moons are for lovers, together or apart. I would never be alone again.

EPILOGUE

It is now 1997, more than sixteen years since I began jotting down material included in this manuscript. At the time my reason for doing so was obvious: I needed to transfer my pain to paper, to fix in my mind the goodness of Monroe, to prevent the wrenching present from destroying what he had meant to me. Without writing I would have given up in despair.

I think I also felt the need to prove to myself and perhaps to others that my grievances were based on reason. Then, as I delved deeper and the indifference or duplicity of Dr. Tarns became more obvious, I came to believe I could never climb the glass mountain the oncology group raised before me because the interests that would rise up to protect Tarns and his institution were stronger than mine. When push came to shove, they would never consider honor a virtue.

Although I have recently learned that Tarns is no longer with the oncology group and has left California, he was still on the staff of the hospital at the time I began writing. That information did nothing to reduce my anger or that of my friends, and I cannot repeat all the forms of mayhem they suggested for him.

"The least you can do," they insisted, "is sue!"

To help me out, a physician friend located the name of a Los Angeles attorney who had won suits against the hospital involved. I phoned this attorney soon after Monroe's final surgery. He explained straight off that the life of an elderly person who has cancer isn't worth much, no matter what the offense against him. He recommended that I take my concerns to the chief administrator of the hospital because the results would be more immediate, and because my intent was to prevent further transgressions rather than to receive money for the injustice done Monroe.

I followed his advice and was, as I wrote earlier, well received by the chief administrator. But I was rebuffed later when I asked to show my evidence to the head of the oncology group and was refused. The form letter response to me turned my desire to be positive into rage and I considered legal action again. But I was only beginning to be rid of the cramps in my gut that had been my daily companions since Monroe's amputation. I knew that a court trial would be painful. I had served on several juries. I knew what an ordeal it was for the families of victims. I had heard their cries of anguish, most of which were sincere; but I had also heard the moans that sounded as though they came on cue from the plaintiff's attorney. The idea of exposing my sorrows in a public court repelled me.

Even so, if I had not been so beaten by the experiences of Monroe's last hospitalization, I might have pulled myself together in time to sue; but I would have had to move fast before the Statute of Limitations ran out on the prime wrongful action I would have stipulated. And, assuming that the time had run out on most of my complaints, would the remaining malfeasance still make legal action worthwhile?

I say "worthwhile" because a suit must be worth the time of a skilled malpractice attorney. Such an attorney does not take a case unless he can expect a large award for his client and for himself. Finding a good attorney is difficult for anyone, let alone for someone involved with a prolonged illness. As long as Monroe was alive, I could not worry him with phone calls about lawsuits and damage done him in the hospital. In Ojai there were no malpractice attorneys, and I could not spare the time away from Monroe to visit a lawyer elsewhere.

Besides, would a lawsuit do anything at all to better the hospital? To make it more responsible and competent? To deal severely with its oncology practitioners?

Even though I doubted it, I could not at the time dismiss the idea of legal action from my mind. I kept on documenting material and writing down information I could give an attorney. I gathered statements from people who had known Monroe well, who had known his behavior both before and after his amputation. I verified names of nurses and checked my notes against hospital statements to make sure that what I said was true. Then, when writing about these experiences became too painful to continue, I wrote down my happy memories of Monroe, dallying the while, not looking hard for a lawyer.

Finally, not long after Monroe died, I located a malpractice attorney in a neighboring city. I asked him to read my manuscript before discussing legal action with me so he would better understand what my grievances were. Over the phone he agreed. But attorneys, too, seem to do things their own way. So, as soon as I sat before his desk, he began, with nary a glance at my manuscript: How old was Monroe? What did the doctor do to kill him? They didn't kill him! Then what's the complaint? He implied that, without death resulting, there was no cause to sue. I tried to draw his attention to my written material, but instead of looking, he announced, "I know you're distraught!"

To which I replied indignantly, "I am not distraught;" and then and there I knew I could never be distraught on cue: that only people who can't control or don't want to control their wailings make a hit in court. I knew that my stomach would rail at acting the piteous plaintiff the attorney would expect of me. I resolved that if I ever went to court, it wouldn't be with him to protect me.

I was glad to escape the attorney's office, but before I left I asked him to obtain the daily notes of the physicians and nurses from the hospital. After they arrived, I incorporated pertinent and often startling revelations into the records I had been keeping. Then I gave a copy of my manuscript with all my evidence to an anesthesiologist friend.

He soon phoned to say he would be a witness if I cared to sue. He thought the legal time had run out on damage done to Monroe's brain in the hospital; but he said I ought to be able to collect a million from the doctors for performing surgery after they had given me false information.

If the amount stated was correct, it should have been worth the while of some attorney; but at the mention of a lawsuit, my gut went into spasm again. Then the anesthesiologist added, "I must say I found your story strangely moving."

His words flowed over me like a benediction. They freed me from further doubt, for if my story could move one physician, might it not move others?

If doctors could only realize that all too often their interventions on hopelessly ill patients are cruel. They are cruel because they do not cure or ease a patient's pain. Instead, they often reduce the quality of a patient's life and leave a family heartbroken, often destitute. According to one physician who has studied health care in both the United States and Europe, European hospitals have "...fewer intensive care units, fewer intensive care patients, and— most dramatically— significantly fewer dying patients."[1]

If doctors could only understand the anguish inflicted on others when they fail to listen, then Monroe's story might serve better than the courts. If technology-dependent health practitioners could understand that reliable observers should never be ignored when a diagnosis and plan of action is made, then my writing would serve better than a lawsuit.

But will physicians change? Can they learn to listen?

A recent clinical study[2] involving more than 8,000 patients was conducted in five highly regarded medical centers. After two years the results showed that more than half of the physicians involved did not know which of their terminally ill patients opposed having their lives extended by invasive equipment. Most of these physicians did not know this in spite of the fact that the patient had a "Do not resuscitate" order entered in the records.

During a second two-year period of this research study, a skilled nurse practitioner worked to ensure that the physicians involved were given accurate information as to the closeness to death of the patients involved plus their written wishes against prolonging their lives by artificial means. Alarmingly, even after special efforts had been made to inform them, the majority of doctors continued to ignore their patients' wishes. They continued to place their patients on machines against their desires and any chance of recovery. The patients died anyway, but their anguish was forcibly continued for a longer period of time.

The results of that study are so negative they depress the hell out of me. Why won't physicians change their ways when faced with compelling evidence that they should?

Is it inertia? That once in motion they continue in a straight line even when it's harmful to the patient?

Is it money? That high tech procedures can't be amortized unless they're used often and long enough?

Is it stupidity, willfulness, heartlessness?

I don't know, but I'm willing to concede that physicians won't change unless and until enough of us become as stubborn and as bullheaded as they.

We must be prepared to communicate our thoughts so firmly that they can't not hear us. And we will have to expect cavalier responses when we do. But I, for one, am tired of being a coward when faced down by the medical profession. I am repelled by the ineptness of my dealings with my husband's physicians. I don't want anything like that to happen again—to me or to anyone else.

I believe we must get clear answers to questions and receive all needed diagnostic information from our physicians.[3] If, for example, I ask my physician how he or she will behave if I am terminally ill and want help in dying as easily as possible, the minimum answer I would accept is that I would be given enough medication to control pain, even if that medicine shortens my life. An answer I would not accept is, "I'll treat you the same as I'd treat my own sister."

What kind of an answer is that? Does he love or hate his sister? Would he honor her wishes? Or would he pat her on the head and extend her life uselessly and painfully, even if she didn't want him to?

Before we undergo a course of treatment or surgery, I believe we should have enough information to compare the procedures proposed. We must know enough to understand what should be expected during recovery and what the odds of success are. This should not be done while we are sedated because our ability to choose wisely will be impaired.

We should also learn if and how our behavior might be affected if we continue to live by means of overly aggressive treatment. Brains of old people are often not able to withstand the trauma of some procedures. If given a choice of possible treatments, we might choose one less effective for prolonging our lives but more likely to not degrade our final days.

Any person, especially an inexperienced woman, trying to level with a condescending physician, might be advised to take along a 6'4" barrel-chested baritone. He might help get the message across. I have often wondered if men do not suffer more and die younger than women because the opinions of their womenfolk are considered by doctors as the brainless assertions of a mother hen.

If we have doubts about a diagnosis or procedure, we should demand a referral. Some insurance companies insist on referral if surgery has been called for.

We have the right to refuse any treatment, and we have the right to leave a hospital without signing a release. This doesn't mean we won't be intimidated. I refused to sign a release for my aged mother from a convalescent hospital until I talked it over with her. The chief administrator overheard my refusal and threatened that my mother would never again be admitted to his hospital if I didn't sign. A year or so later my mother was readmitted to that hospital even though I had refused to toady to him.

All too often the only way to protect the ones we love from procedures we do not want is to take them out of the hospital. Only recently a friend told me that her husband's physicians and their hospital refused to comply even though she held her husband's Durable Power of Attorney for Health Care Decisions. He had written his opposition to artificial life supports. She had to take him home where he could die in dignity and without machines to prolong his life. Needless to say, she was traumatized by the obstacles the doctors threw in her way at a time when she needed support, not abuse.

One of the things for which I am most grateful is that I could keep Monroe at home and away from the hassles of a hospital during the last two years of his life. We both suffered less in the familiarity and tranquility of our own home. We both gained peace. But I know that not everyone can do what I did. Not everyone has adequate home facilities and a caretaker with enough physical strength to handle the problems.

Just as we have the right to leave a hospital, we have the right to stay in it if we can't cope otherwise. (But our insurance company may have the right to refuse to pay for extended time.) We have the right to all of our medical records. I paid an attorney to get my husband's records for me because I didn't know that a lawyer wasn't necessary. We also have the right to be informed of what we will need to do and have on hand after leaving the hospital. I was well within my right to keep Monroe in the hospital when I had not been trained to bind his stump.

It is extremely important to know how our physicians obtain their earned income. Our health care practitioner may be self-employed, salaried, or largely dependent on bonuses paid by an insurance company for holding costs down. If it is the latter, beware, because a physician who accepts a reward for not ordering an appropriate procedure can hardly be offering good health care. My own main drive and concerns, quite obviously, have been with over-use of medicines and equipment, but I certainly do not advocate saving money at the expense of good health care.

Lastly, we do have the right to deny information about our health condition to anyone. But, unless there is a strong reason to the contrary, it is usually not wise to keep knowledge of our impending death from family members. It is usually kinder to let them know, to communicate sincerely with them. Foreknowledge allows for reconciliation with death and with each other.

One night when we were young, Monroe was listening as I read a fairy tale to our son. Throughout the story ran the reassuring refrain, "I shall never forsake you if you never forsake me." The words were repeated so often that Monroe began to laugh, and so did I. The sentence became a family slogan. Whenever I was down, Monroe would say, "Don't worry. I shall never forsake you if you never forsake me." It always made me giggle.

Years later, when life became so bleak I could no longer understand the man I loved, I was twice advised to leave him. But if I had forsaken him and learned the truth too late, my remorse would have devoured me.

But I did not forsake him because I learned the truth in time. I learned it despite the secrecy, indifference, and neglect of the physicians he trusted. And I learned it in time to break the tangles of misunderstanding that had grown between Monroe and me.

For that I am forever grateful.

ENDNOTES

1 **Academic Medicine,** "Cost Containment in U.S. Health Care," No. 10, October, 1995, Vol.70.

2 **Journal of the American Medical Association**, "A Controlled Trial to Improve Care for Seriously Ill Hospitalized Patients: The Study to Understand Prognoses and Preference for Outcomes and Risks of Treatment (SUPPORT)," Nov. 22/29, 1995, Vol. 274.

3 These "rules" in the text are borrowed largely from "Patients Rights and Resources" compiled by the Hemlock Society, USA, Denver, Colorado. (The comments and asides are my own).

ORDER FORM

Pathfinder Publishing of California
458 Dorothy Ave.
Ventura, CA 93003-1723

Telephone (805) 642-9278   FAX (805) 650-3656
Book Order Telephone Line: (800) 977-2282

Please send me the following books from Pathfinder Publishing:

_____Copies of **Beyond Sympathy** @ $11.95 $_____
_____Copies of **Injury** @ $9.95 $_____
_____Copies of **In Search of My Husband's Mind** @$22.00 $_____
_____Copies of **Living Creatively**
                    With Chronic Illness @ $11.95 $_____
_____Copies of **Managing Your Health Care** @ $9.95 $_____
_____Copies of **No Time For Goodbyes** @ $11.95 $_____
_____Copies of **Quest For Respect** @ $9.95 $_____
_____Copies of **Sexual Challenges** @ $11.95 $_____
_____Copies of **Surviving an Auto Accident** @ $9.95 $_____
_____Copies of **Violence in our Schools, Hospitals and**
                    Public Places   @ $22.95 Hard Cover $_____
_____   @ $14.95 Soft Cover $_____
_____Copies of **Violence in the Workplace** @ $22.95 Hard $_____
                    Violence in the Workplace @ $14.95 Soft $_____
_____Copies of **When There Are No Words** @ $9.95 $_____
                                                    Sub-Total $_____
                    Californians: Please add 7.25% tax. $_____
                    Shipping* $_____
                                                    Grand Total $_____

I understand that I may return the book for a full refund if not satisfied.
Name:_____

Address:_____
_____ ZIP:_____

*SHIPPING CHARGES U.S.
Books: Enclose $3.25 for the first book and .50c for each additional
book. UPS: Truck; $4.50 for first item, .50c for each additional. UPS
2nd Day Air: $10.75 for first item, $1.00 for each additional item.
Master and Visa Credit Cards orders are acceptable.